Sick Girl Speaks!

Sick Girl Speaks!

Lessons and Ponderings Along the Road to Acceptance

Tiffany Christensen

iUniverse, Inc.
New York Lincoln Shanghai

Sick Girl Speaks!
Lessons and Ponderings Along the Road to Acceptance

iUniverse books may be ordered through booksellers or by contacting:

iUniverse
2021 Pine Lake Road, Suite 100
Lincoln, NE 68512
www.iuniverse.com
1-800-Authors (1-800-288-4677)

Because of the dynamic nature of the Internet, any Web addresses
or links contained in this book may have changed
since publication and may no longer be valid.

The views expressed in this work are solely those of the author and do not
necessarily reflect the views of the publisher, and the publisher hereby
disclaims any responsibility for them.

ISBN: 978-0-595-47201-7 (pbk)
ISBN: 978-0-595-91611-5 (cloth)
ISBN: 978-0-595-91482-1 (ebk)

Printed in the United States of America

This book is dedicated to the late Treya Wilber
She led a dynamic life and died an admirable death

Her example of strength, insight and balance has shown me
a better way to live and to die

Contents

Still Not Dead

Most of us will become ill at some point in our lifetime. Many of us will find ourselves in the medical system, either as a patient or caregiver. For patients and families, the world of medicine can be disorienting and difficult.

I was born with cystic fibrosis and have undergone two double lung transplant surgeries. Despite that, this is not a book about transplant or CF. In my travels, I've had the opportunity to interact with many patients with a wide variety of diagnoses. While we may have been on different medications, had different surgeries or experienced different symptoms, the emotional, spiritual and psychological effects were often nearly identical.

I was inspired to write this book after a conversation with a friend who came to visit me one summer. Her father had just had a stroke and was in the hospital. She told stories filled with fear and sadness because she was so lost in the medical maze while desperately trying to take good care of her dad. I was overwhelmed with the desire to share with her all that I had learned through the years of stumbling through my own illness maze.

Those of us who enter the medical maze usually find ourselves hitting more than one or two walls. Those walls are invariably emotional as well as physical. There are countless ways to cope, some of them healthy, some of them destructive. A modern theme that is emerging is the desire to control illness using diet, exercise and positive thinking. The traditional approach is, of course, Western medicine for all of what ails you, even the fear and sadness part. For every person with illness, there are countless belief systems and approaches to treatment for them to explore.

While different schools of thought debate one another, the theme in my life has become quite clear. I "battle" my illnesses with acceptance. Of the perspectives I have entertained, I find very few to be entirely flawed. I have not found any to be perfect. What I know now is that acceptance is the only thing that will bring peace into my life, no matter what happens to me physically.

If I become attached to a certain medication or thought pattern, becoming convinced that it will eliminate illness from my life, chances are, I will be devastated over and over. At the core, I know that *I am not illness*. My body, however, is bound to different rules and is not something I can always control or manipulate into wellness. If I allow room in my heart for a new treatment but remain calm in knowing that things might get better, they might get worse or they could stay the same, I can never be hurt by the unpredictable nature of physical illness.

With all of that said, illness is not a theoretical concept. It is a real circumstance that can be approached mindfully or unconsciously. Dealing with doctors and hospitals can be frustrating and frightening. I have tried to include concrete, practical parts to this book so that patients and families might navigate more effectively and with more confidence within the medical maze. It is my hope that providing some tips and tricks will help someone bypass painful obstacles that I ran into headfirst and had to overcome the hard way.

In addition to the practical tips in this book, I've taken my personal journals off of the shelf, dusted them off, and transcribed them. Although I feel quite vulnerable exposing these entries, I believe it's important to open the door into the private thoughts and emotions of a person facing illness. I offer my journals as an affirmation; there will be times of sorrow and times of joy on everyone's path—both of those are okay, even "normal." I imagine many who read my emotional confessions will see themselves in the writing.

Another aspect of this book is my ponderings related to the spiritual side of illness. I speak of God and make other "religious" references. I struggled with my decision to include this aspect of my life in this book. These days, it's so easy to turn people away by using a religious reference that isn't in sync with their own. In the end, I couldn't leave out my relationship with the divine; it was a huge part of my experience. I've found great inspiration and clarity through many different religions, and ultimately found that one's intention is what's most important. I hope my language and personal choices about spiritual issues won't be a distraction from my intention.

Last, but certainly not least, I've written this book for professional caregivers. Throughout my illness journey, I've been surprised to discover that many doctors and nurses lack a real understanding of the patient experience. I also found many of them truly desire that insight but don't know where to find it. Well, now they can find it right here.

It is important that I share with you some of my history so that you might understand how my experiences influence the perspectives in this book. You will see, there are lots of reasons that I should be dead by now! Few people have logged as many hours in the hospital as I have, and lived to talk about it. I don't see this as a burden but a privilege. For this reason, I feel it is my duty to speak up about what I have seen and done.

I was born with cystic fibrosis, a genetic illness that affects the lungs and digestion. In 1973, the year I came into this body, the life expectancy for a person with CF was around eight. As medicine advanced, I seemed to stay right behind that number. When I was eight, the number was twelve. When I was twelve, the number was twenty-one, and so on.

I had countless bouts of pneumonia and bronchitis growing up. A few times I was so sick my mother had a minister in to bless me in case I died. I managed to graduate from high school in between trips to the hospital, and I went on to college. At that point, I was so chronically ill that I was getting powerful intravenous antibiotics every few weeks, for weeks at a time. If you do the math, that means there were rarely times when I was *not* getting IV medication. Not surprisingly, my health ran out before I could graduate. I left college and the doctors put me on the lung transplant list. My health was failing and that was my only hope for survival.

I waited five years for my first transplant, getting sicker and sicker. I had to carry oxygen with me twenty-four hours a day. I couldn't work and needed plenty of help to manage average tasks. I was dying.

On April 4, 2000 I got the call: they might have lungs for me. My family and I drove to the hospital, excited and terrified. There was the excitement that I may live a life in which breathing came easily. There was the fear the surgery would be too much for my body and I'd never make it home again. In my heart, I believed I'd make it through the operation and do well.

I spent a month in the hospital with various complications, my recovery slow and difficult. But, once I was able to run around, I didn't want to stop. For the first time since I was born, I could breathe deeply. I devoured life with a ravenous appetite. My hunger was so disorienting, it was impossible for me to pick a direction or path. I was all over the map for months until, like hitting a brick wall, a medicine-induced depression hit me. I spent the next eight months in a deep hole, wondering what the point was of my life being saved. I eventually emerged, but had no better compass for what direction I should choose for my life.

Ultimately, I chose to go back to school. I was enjoying it and beginning to think I might have a worthwhile future ahead. Twenty-six months after my transplant, I was given horrible news. I'd developed chronic rejection, a puzzling and devastating illness with very few treatment possibilities. My lung function took a steady dive downwards and never really stopped. I had to quit school again, and reorganize my life for this new and uninvited guest. After a year, I was back on oxygen, already quite enfeebled.

Just when I was beginning to find my place in this life, I was dying again. I asked my medical team if they would consider giving me another lung transplant. They declined, saying it was too risky and rarely successful. My options had run out and I had to say goodbye.

I rode the roller coaster of emotions, all the ones outlined by Kubler-Ross, over and over again. Grief isn't a linear process, and I experienced denial, anger, sadness, bargaining and acceptance in many different shapes and forms. I did eventually land in the soft bed of acceptance. I had faced my mortality, grieved my losses, and found beauty in my terminal illness. I was truly at peace.

That peace was unexpectedly interrupted by my earth angel, the new transplant coordinator. When she heard I'd expressed an interest in a second transplant, something in her was motivated to give me that chance. She wanted to find a way to put me on the list again.

My initial reaction wasn't one of joy. I was a jumble of anger, hope and dread, with a large dose of confusion. I'd made peace with my fate and now I had to consider the possibility of living? This seemed far more difficult than simply accepting death.

In 2004, I did get another transplant. My health, while still having a few bumps here and there, has been extraordinary. As a person who's lived with acute illness, chronic illness, sudden-onset illness and terminal illness, I have much to be grateful for.

There's a saying: "To whom much has been given, much is expected." All of the procedures, medicines and surgeries my body has endured are mind-boggling. I strive to live my life boldly and passionately while I still have the health to do so. Along the way, I hope that my efforts will be an offering to those I love and those who saved my life, both the medical staff and my donors. I have much to share and still much to learn. By the grace of God and with the help of many beloved people, I'm still not dead.

The Medical Maze

It's time for a medical revolution.

The time has come to let go of past perceptions and move forward into the age of patient empowerment!

Patients, let's break down those archaic ideas about doctors having all the answers and learn to become proactive in our life and our care.

Professionals, let's stop treating patients like helpless children and work to create a partnership, rather than a dictatorship, in care giving.

There's much room to grow on both sides of the medical fence.

Squeaky Wheel

A good doctor will make you feel as though you're the only patient they have. A bad doctor will make you feel like a complete inconvenience to their day. The truth lies somewhere in between.

Worry and Wait:

A friend went in to see her specialist complaining of numbness in her legs, extreme fatigue and strange tingling sensations up and down her left side. Casually, the doctor mentioned that it could be multiple sclerosis, among other possibilities. Because her mother has MS, it was obviously the possibility that stuck out in her mind and sent chills of fear through her aching bones.

They took blood and promised the results would be back on Friday, four days later. Four very long, scary and uncomfortable days. During that time her symptoms grew worse and she began to have additional ones, the primary being painful white bumps on the back of her throat.

Thursday came and went with no call about her test results. At my urging, she decided to be a "squeaky wheel" and call before the end of business on Friday with two objectives: to see if her blood-work results had come in and to offer up her new symptoms since they might be a key in figuring out what she was dealing with.

She called at two o'clock and the office had already closed at one. Choosing to go against her instinct to be "nice" and wait until Monday, she called the emergency number given. Surprisingly, the doctor himself answered the phone. She began to tell him her newest symptoms and he gave her a quick over-the-phone diagnosis. Before she could ask what her blood work showed or if the new symptoms were related, he had another call and had to get off the phone immediately. She held on the line, waiting for him to finish the other call, only to be met with an impatient click and "What else do you want?" She could barely get any words out before he again claimed the urgency of the other call and hung up. Naively, my friend thought he'd call back. He didn't.

At some point it dawned on her he may not have even remembered her case and the fact that he'd said she may have multiple sclerosis. He thought she was calling the emergency line about white bumps in the back of her throat!

Had it been me, I like to think I'd have called him again, but I can't be sure of that. For people who aren't used to or comfortable with being assertive, it's often very difficult to push an issue with the medical team. For my friend, calling the emergency number was a bold move and calling it again seemed out of the question. She spent the rest of her weekend being very sick with no idea what was happening to her. For the doctor, it was just two more days. For a patient, it's a lifetime of worry and contemplation.

What You Don't Know Can Hurt You:

The same friend I wrote about in the previous story went into the hospital with a painful kidney infection. She was on intravenous antibiotics and fluids. Somewhere between the antibiotics and the illness itself, she was intensely nauseous. Every time a nurse or doctor asked how she was doing she mentioned this problem. They gave her a look of sympathy and moved on to the next question.

When she and I spoke on the phone I asked her why they hadn't given her any anti-nausea meds. She didn't even know such a thing existed!

She buzzed the nurse, told her she'd like some anti-nausea meds and within an hour she was given something. Her relief was evident in her voice and she asked me why nobody had mentioned that possibility to her.

I really don't understand this, but often you must ask the *direct question* "Is there anything you can give me to help me with this symptom?" before you're given the option. In fact, there are many anti-nausea medications, and it took me years to learn that I preferred an alternative to the one I was commonly given. There's another one that works much better for me and I now always specify when I'm getting anti-nausea medications. Not only must you squeak enough to find out if there's relief available but you also must explore the various options for that relief.

Dying Again?:

Two years after my second transplant, I had a drop in my pulmonary function. The doctors became very concerned and ordered a bronchoscopy immediately. What followed were intravenous steroids, more immunosuppressant drugs and my third terminal diagnosis. They said I had chronic rejection again, the illness that had almost killed me only two years earlier. I was devastated. I began to plan for my life in the sick world, and revisited what it was to "die well."

During this time, my doctors seemed to be having trouble agreeing on my treatment. Some wanted to try more steroids; some voted for a form of chemotherapy; some had the wait-and-see approach. The chemotherapy option was a concern; it meant feeling poorly and being hospitalized. I needed a decision urgently as I would need to schedule time off from work, get ready to be an in-patient and emotionally prepare for chemo. I went a week with no answer on the next step.

Finally, I went in to the clinic, hoping my physical presence would prompt a decision. That didn't work, but an answer was promised by the end of the day, and it was a Friday. At three I started calling my transplant coordinator, and I called every half hour. When she returned my call she said I was "fine." Apparently, the team had decided to do nothing as they no longer thought I had chronic rejection. She was astounded I hadn't already heard this news. My reaction wasn't one of sheer happiness, as you might expect. I was confused.

As it turned out I'd been prematurely diagnosed, and I didn't need more steroids or chemotherapy. Of course, I was relieved after the shock wore off, but I'm still amazed by that series of events. It became clear to me that there are times when little consideration is given to the mental or emotional state of patients waiting for life-changing news.

What I Know Now:

As a patient, I've learned the value of being a squeaky wheel. As someone who works in a doctor's office, I've learned the necessity of being a squeaky wheel.

You're one of many, many people a doctor sees during the course of a day. Unless your case is incredibly unusual or acute, it's very unlikely you'll be at the front of their mind. They will revisit your case only when the lab work returns (for example) and it might take some time to refresh their memory. If you aren't "bothering" them, you're much more likely to be put at the bottom of the stack. That can mean a long weekend of worry, unattended discomfort, or possibly even worse.

There's a fine line between being a squeaky wheel and being a pain-in-the-butt that will make people not want to help you. Don't assume they're putting themselves in your shoes. Don't assume they're thinking about you at all. At the same time, don't allow yourself to be so arrogant as to assume you always know more than your health care team. Be aware they may have methods that you don't understand. I like to qualify it by saying you must be a *humble, polite, persistent* squeaky wheel.

Fight for your information without alienating the team. Don't be afraid to be that squeaky wheel so you will get the best care possible!

Top 10 *Actual* Quotes from Medical Professionals
(that made me want to run screaming from the room)

1. "It's been a long time since I've dealt with real patients."

2. Her: "You have good veins, right?" Me: "No." Her (sarcastically): "Oh, grrrreeeat!"

3. "How do you spell cystic?"

4. "Let me go ask what this test is."

5. "I don't remember our conversation about you medication allergies. I was on pain meds."

6. "Did you pass gas from your bottom?"

7. "You don't have any pain medication ordered so you can't have any."

8. "Oooh, we didn't realize you had *that* procedure done. We'll need to run that test again."

9. "Ewww. Gross. Your urine smells like cat pee."

10. "I hate this f***ing rotation!" (spoken while cutting my arm open to place a PIC line)

Choosing Your Doctor

Here's the truth: Your care is only as good as the doctor in charge of it. You may be at one of the best medical facilities in the country but that's no guarantee. Certainly, that increases your odds of getting a good doctor but it's still a role of the dice. At the same time, you may be at a small hospital in the middle of nowhere and find yourself a real gem.

Did you know that you could choose your doctor? Not many people do. You can and you should! It's your job to evaluate the care your doctor is giving you. The question is: How do you know which one to pick?

Discouraging Words:

When I was twenty-one, I had a doctor who was treating me for CF. I was in college, but struggling to stay in as my health was deteriorating. Amazingly, nobody had ever mentioned transplant to me. For all I knew my life was going to be a series of lung infections, IV therapy and feeling the way I had always felt.

This doctor made comments to me I'll never forget. He told me my health was "pathetic" and that he often sees CF women hit twenty-one and "go downhill." He casually told me I needed a transplant, and it was as though a bucket of cold water had been thrown in my face.

Looking back, I see he knew things I didn't know: this was a trend and the changes in my health were normal. Looking back, I wonder if perhaps he was actually a well-informed doctor who knew what he was doing.

I also see that "transplant" is just another word in the vocabulary of a CF doctor, and it wasn't his intention to terrify me. But he did. I imagine he didn't understand the pain and fear that his words roused in me.

I also know that, had he thought about my position, he could have helped me understand my current health was expected, a typical course for someone like me, and he could have given me options to think about. He could have made me feel good about transplant and my hope for the future.

I can see now that he had a tremendous opportunity to inspire me, but instead I fired him and wouldn't let anyone mention the word transplant for an entire year. He could have done his job differently and changed the course of my life.

Maybe he was uncomfortable with giving me bad news. Maybe he'd forgotten that I was a person and not just a grouping of cells and genetics. Whatever his reason for speaking to me the way he did it made me seek a way out of his care.

At some point, I had to be admitted into the hospital for a tune-up. Luckily for me, he wasn't the doctor assigned to the floor that month. A wonderful, sweet man was taking care of me and I very much wished he would be my doctor. One day, like a young boy asking out his dream girl, I asked this doctor if he'd take over my care after my hospital stay.

To my delight, his response was "Of course." The next day I asked to see the original doctor and he came by my room. I handed him a book that was popular at the time that explored the mind/body connection. I calmly explained why I no longer wanted him as my doctor. He wasn't surprised. His own wife had told him that he shouldn't be working with patients! I was told that soon after our talk, he went into research.

Meanwhile, I became the patient of a wonderful doctor who took great care of me for many, many years. Since he left the area, I've had other doctors—some of whom I kept, some of whom I fired.

Forgotten and Not Forgiven:

I was being treated at a California University hospital and there was only one man in the CF department. I quite liked him and was happy to have him as my doctor. Over time, I found things I didn't like, but continued under his care anyway.

At some point, he needed to go into the hospital for a minor surgery. At that same time, I was very sick and needed to be admitted for IV antibiotics. I spoke with him directly and was sure to remind him not to prescribe a certain IV antibiotic since it makes me extremely sick. He agreed and I checked into the hospital. In the middle of the night I awoke and began to violently vomit. I managed to look at the IV bag hanging beside my bed and saw he had prescribed the exact medication we had just discussed avoiding. The nurse had hung it while I was asleep so I hadn't been able to check it first. I was furious.

When he came in for morning rounds I asked him why he had done such a thing. His response was that he had been on pain meds from his surgery and didn't really remember our conversation. This is the downside to individual care. When you're the only doctor, it's difficult to take time off, and when you're the unhappy patient, there's nowhere within the system to turn. I left his care and went to another California University hospital that was based on the team approach.

What I Know Now:

Compatibility with your doctor is an issue of great importance. Whether you see him or her once a year or once a week, it's important to have some of the same philosophies and approaches to your health care.

Personality is important, and that's obviously something completely unique in every situation. There are, however, a few generalizations I can make about doctors that are worth considering when deciding if you and your doc are a good match. At the very least, it's imperative to know that when it comes to your main physician, you do have choices.

Individual vs. Team

Both of these options have clear pros and cons. Being treated by an individual allows more room for consistency and personal interaction. For the most part, I find this to be ideal. However, the above example is one dramatic experience that can outline the flaw in this system of care.

The upside of the team approach is that there are many doctors working with you who are able to put their heads together to find the course of care best for you. There's less burnout and there's always someone to cover for a sick or otherwise unavailable doctor.

The down-side of the team approach is the revolving door. Each time I go to clinic at my Carolina hospital I seem to have a different doctor. There's less consistency of care and less of a personal rapport. Sometimes, the team doesn't agree on the next step and this can cause a gridlock that will postpone your treatment for days, maybe even weeks.

Conservative vs. Laid Back

By conservative, I don't mean politically. There are some doctors who won't take a chance with your health in any way. That means, if you come in with a fever, they'll send you for blood-work, a CAT scan and urinalysis before they're satisfied you only have a passing virus. The laid back doctor, however, will assume it's nothing before they assume it's anything. They'll send you home and let the presumed virus run its course before they'll order tests or prescribe meds. Both have pros and cons, but it's important to know which approach you prefer before choosing a doctor.

Old vs. Young

At the risk of being ageist, I've found there are general differences in the two. They both have very distinct benefits and it's up to you to decide which ones seem more important.

An older doctor obviously has more experience. For the patient this translates into less guess work and unnecessary tests. I've often gone in to see an older doctor with unusual symptoms and they know right away what's wrong with me. Why? Because they've seen it first-hand many times before. During times of crisis, I often breathe a sigh of relief when I see the white-haired physician enter my room!

A younger doctor may have to do a little more research to figure out the cause of your problems, but is more often up on all the latest drugs and technologies. Medicine changes rapidly, and it's difficult to keep up. A younger doctor is more likely to know about a new procedure or treatment that can be a smoother road for you than the roads of yesteryear. When I see my doctor pull out a pocket computer it warms my heart!

Male vs. Female

The difference between male and female doctors is very much what you might expect. Women tend to be better at the whole beside manner thing. I've no evidence to suggest they're better or worse doctors than men, but I do sometimes worry that their emotionality can lead to a quicker burn-out.

Current Philosophy

In many areas of medicine, there's a drive to use the latest and greatest theories to enhance or prolong life. What's interesting is that no two centers seem to have the same idea of what that "latest and greatest" may be.

When I was waiting for my first set of donor lungs I moved to California. I was very sick but I figured I could wait somewhere new, different and warm—as opposed to the third floor bedroom at my parents' townhouse. I transferred my care to a California University medical center but I was still considered a patient of Carolina University. Because of this, I wasn't bound by the philosophies of California.

At that time, all California CF lung transplant patients were required to undergo sinus surgery before the transplant. The theory behind this was that the sinuses harbored infection and that infection could eventually infect the new lungs, and, therefore, it was best to clean them out. My doctor at home completely disagreed with that idea. He felt strongly that many patients would die while having the sinus surgery and was far too great of a risk to take.

This kind of disagreement with procedures isn't at all uncommon. Medical theories and practices change with the wind, and when you're choosing your doctor, you may also be choosing a certain protocol. Be sure to do your research and discover for yourself if this is a protocol you agree with.

Utopian Hospital

Journal entry from December, 2000

Holy Moly Guacamole! I always forget what an annoying mess it is to be in the hospital—that is, until I return. It's been about a year since I've been in-house but all of the memories are flooding back to me now.

I woke up yesterday morning to the usual—a phlebotomist turning on the overhead florescent light and preparing to pull out enough blood to make my veins run dry. I did my usual: asking which tests she was drawing for. Of course, she said she was there to draw my tac level.

Side Note: Tac is short for Tacrolimus and is the main immunosuppressant used to keep my lungs from rejecting. It is necessary to test the blood to make sure the drug level is high enough to be effective but not too high as it can be toxic. This kind of test is called a peak and trough and must be done at the correct time— usually twelve hours after the drug has been given.

Here's the thing—it was too early for the test. You know what that means! The test will be useless but the doctors will see the results, freak out and up my dose. I tried to explain this to the phlebotomist but she wasn't having it. She insisted on drawing my blood and I suggested she get her schedule straight. She got really angry with me and went to find my nurse.

The nurse came in, visibly flustered, and assured me that it would be fine to draw the blood despite the time. I knew she was wrong but I let them do it anyway. It was way too early for all that arguing and, anyway, there were other tests to be done.

Sure enough, when the team rounded they told me that my tac levels were too low and they wanted to bump me up. I tried to explain what happened but I'm not dealing with transplant doctors and they really don't seem to understand the importance of the timing on a peak and trough.

This morning, it was the same song and dance but, this time, they drew the blood after I had already taken my meds. Right on cue the docs came in with their hair on fire. Apparently my tac level was through the roof and my blood sugar was even higher. I try to explain that they drew my blood at the wrong time and so it was an inaccurate test. I also pointed out that today is a prednisone day which often makes my blood sugar much higher.

The Queen Resident didn't appreciate my teaching session and she gave me all kinds of attitude. Man, that woman thinks she knows *everything*! It took a long time for me to convince them that everything was really okay.

This is a minor example of the major annoying stuff that happens every day in this place. After awhile, you get used to it and learn how to prevent and put out fires. Nonetheless, it never really stops being irritating.

I have designed a utopian hospital in my head. In my world, hospitals would be far more organized, for starters. There wouldn't be all these silly miscommunications and doctors would consult with patients, not rule over them.

Beyond that, hospitals would be prettier and every window would have a great view. The IV machines would not be equipped with that horrible beeping noise, but, instead, send a silent message to the nurse's station. The food would be nourishing and delicious. There would be massage therapists on staff to help with the aches and pains of lying in bed. There would be yoga classes down the hall and Jacuzzi tubs to bathe in. There would be one nurse for every two patients so whenever I needed nausea or pain meds I would have them right away. There would be soft carpeting under my feet and the beds would be cozy and comfortable. At night, it would be quiet and dark and I would sleep like a baby.

In my utopian hospital, an equal emphasis would be placed on healing as there is on medicating the body. Rest and nourishment would be as important as getting the correct antibiotics. When I walked into the hospital, I would look forward to being taken care of instead of being on guard. I would leave feeling refreshed rather than worn down, hungry and exhausted.

In the meantime, here I sit, like a watch dog, waiting for my next encounter with a stranger. I am so tired.

Getting Your PhD in Patientology

I'm sorry to be the one to break the news: Gone are the days when doctors know all and we're at their mercy. When it comes to your personal care, it's your job to gather all the information you can on the consequences of different procedures, your medications and your own body. That's not a suggestion, it's a necessity, and could save your life.

As a patient, the world of medicine is intimidating. There's a lot to learn and retain. You never know when a tidbit of information is going to play a key part in your medical drama. While you may not have the medical degree you are, in many respects, the most qualified expert in the room. You know your body and your history better than anyone else and it's to your benefit to assert your role as expert.

Good medical professionals will come and go from your life. Make sure that you have enough understanding of your needs that a few not-so-good medical professionals won't prevent you from getting the care you require.

The Road to Confusion is Paved with Post-it Notes:

There was a time when I had a transplant coordinator named Betty, who left much to be desired. She primarily organized her patients' care with post-it notes and always chose the path that required the least amount of work for her.

I was on a downward spiral after recently being diagnosed with chronic rejection. My lung function was dropping almost daily and the doctors were struggling to get me stabilized. In addition, I was having persistent fevers that were concerning because if my body's immune responses were too high, I could also go into another form of rejection called acute rejection.

I went to clinic to address the fevers and was seen by a doctor who hadn't been on the team long, and, in the end, didn't stay long either. His analysis was that the fevers were being caused by chronic sinus infections and his solution was sinus surgery.

Based on his conclusion, the wheels began turning to set me up for the surgery. I saw the ENT doctor and he felt, based on my history, it would be a good idea to do the surgery, but not a necessity. We went forward and made the surgery appointment.

The day before I was to go in, I had to go into the hospital for a battery of pre-surgery tests. I had one question on my mind that had never been answered: If my lung function was continuing to drop, wouldn't being intubated and going under anesthesia make that problem worse? I knew intubation and anesthesia were difficult to recover from when one was having lung issues.

The tests I had to have done took all day and were at a variety of different places throughout the hospital. At each stop I asked the caregiver when I'd be able to see a doctor and ask them my question. The answer was always "later." Finally, at nearly five p.m., I was at the final stop. I asked the nurse my question, and, for the first time that day, her response was one of concern. She felt I had a valid question and encouraged me to contact my transplant coordinator. She gave me a phone and I called.

Betty answered, to my surprise, and I told her my thoughts. She exclaimed that she had a note on her desk to call me. At some point, she had realized I shouldn't have the sinus surgery until my lung function had stabilized. I reminded her I was only hours away from going under anesthesia. She said she simply hadn't gotten around to contacting me yet.

After we hung up, the surgery was canceled and I went home. What if I hadn't been paying attention when someone mentioned the effects of general anesthesia on lung function? What if I had undergone the surgery and Betty got around to calling me *afterwards*? We will never know. I'm just glad I remembered the anesthesia issue and pushed for an answer.

In the end, my fevers resolved and I never did have the sinus surgery.

No Detail Too Small:

After transplant, there are many, many medications a patient has to take. Some of them have side effects and some of them are counter-indicated. For instance, the major immunosuppressant can't be taken with any ibuprofen product because the two together can cause kidney failure. This is something they try to teach you when you're learning your medications, but a friend of mine missed that lesson.

After his surgery, he was having back pain and began to take ibuprofen to help. A few days later, his lower back began to hurt and the pain extended all the way down the back of his thighs. Fortunately, he mentioned this at a clinic visit and it was quickly discovered he was in early-stage renal failure. They were able to treat him and reverse the effects of the ibuprofen interaction, but he was shaken.

This wasn't the fault of the doctors or nurses. My friend failed to take in crucial information that was provided to him. It can be easy to become complacent with your care and not think about all the details. That approach can clearly lead to a world of trouble.

Fear and Trembling, I Promise:

I like to think of myself as a unique individual, but, when it comes to my body, that isn't really a compliment. I can react to things very differently than most people. Some of that has to do with my emotional history; some has to do with my varying pain tolerance; and some has to do with my personal body chemistry. Only I can know how I will handle certain medications and procedures, and I have to somehow find ways to communicate these idiosyncrasies to those caring for me.

At one point, I had a central line called a Port-a-Catheter. This was a wonderful device that allowed me to get IV medications with minimal pain and was far less invasive than having an IV in my arm. After my first transplant, this catheter was taken out since it posed a risk of infection. From that point on, I required a PIC line whenever I needed IV medications. This catheter is placed above the elbow and is fed in across the chest, stopping just short of the heart. For most people, apparently, this is no big deal. For me it's incredibly painful. Between the existing scar tissue from past blood draws and IV catheters and the fact that I'm very small, this procedure is at the top of my Most-hated Procedures list.

When it comes to getting a PIC line placed, I've become a Pavlovian dog. As soon as they wheel me into the room where it's done I start to feel cold, tremble and cry uncontrollably. This isn't a welcoming sight to those involved in doing the procedure and makes it all the more traumatic for me. At times I've even had this reaction when I'm simply filling out the paperwork.

There have been doctors who gave me PIC lines that felt compassion for me. There have been doctors who've told me I shouldn't be so upset. There have been doctors who did it very well and it turned out to be not so bad. There were doctors who did it very forcefully and I was in terrible pain for days afterwards. No matter what the circumstances, my reaction remains the same; I'm scarred for life when it comes to PIC lines.

So what do I do? It's my job to convince them of the severity of my problem and make sure that I'm provided with the proper pre-medication. I need to be very sedated before I go in that room. It can take time to convince someone that I *need* this pre-medication since that's not a normal request. Eventually, I may have to declare that I won't do it without the sedation. If that doesn't work, it's then necessary to involve my transplant doctors in the debate. Usually, it doesn't come to that, but, regardless, I won't back down from this demand. It's my body and I know it better than anyone else. End of story.

What I Know Now:

Everyone knows that knowledge is power. In this case, knowledge can come in the form of medical details or a personal understanding of your own body's needs. When it comes to health care, it can enhance or even save your life. The more you can learn about your illness and the treatments, the better able you'll be to make informed decisions and ask the right questions. The more you pay attention and document the physical reactions you experience, the better able you will be to advocate for solutions to problems that are unique to you.

Information can be gathered from other patients, the internet, reading books and asking lots and lots of questions to the medical professionals around you. Take control. Knowledge is the first key in being an effective patient advocate.

Awareness and Boundaries

No matter which hospital you go to or which doctor you see, the potential for mistakes is simply a reality that can't be ignored. In 2006, it was reported that medical mistakes are responsible for about 250 deaths a day.

I can't help but wonder how many of those mistakes could have been avoided if patients were more pro-active in their care. With knowledge being the first key in protecting yourself in a medical setting, awareness and boundaries are close behind.

I Know What I Know So—No!:

I wish I could be more technical about this example. Don't let the fact that I can't remember the exact name of the medication make you doubt the validity of this event. I promise, it's true.

When I was in the hospital after lung transplant number one, I was receiving injections. I can't remember why, or, again, what the name of the medication was. What I do remember is that my nurse told me I should only get this injection once a day. As she administered it, she stressed this to me and I remembered.

One evening, right after shift change, another nurse came in with a syringe. She told me it was time for the injection. I immediately protested that I'd already received that dose for the day. This nurse absolutely didn't believe me. After all, I was the one taking high-powered narcotics, right?

At my insistence, she rechecked the chart and reported that it hadn't been noted, and, therefore, it *hadn't* been done. I was adamant that it had and insisted she call the previous nurse at home. I was walking a thin line and she was getting irritated. Nonetheless, she followed through and left my room to make the call.

Minutes later, she came back in, her face quite flushed. She apologized profusely and acknowledged that I had, indeed, had the injection earlier that day.

The previous nurse had confirmed this and was mortified that she hadn't marked it in the chart.

With her hands a little shaky, the evening nurse put her hand on my knee and whispered, "It could have killed you." I smiled, and was very proud of myself. I'd successfully been aware of what medications I'd been given that day and, ultimately, had been equally successful in setting up proper boundaries that saved me from great distress.

Protecting the Final Two:

Of all the procedures I've ever had done, blood draws have been the most common and numerous. Unfortunately, because of all of the IVs and needle pokes I've had in my life, I only have two veins left that can be used to take blood. They're both in my right hand.

These veins are extremely valuable to me and I guard them like a vicious watch dog. When I walk into the lab or wake up to a phlebotomist in the hospital, I know they don't understand my history or how precious those veins are. It's my job to set boundaries to ensure they don't get blown or otherwise badly scarred.

I immediately establish with the phlebotomist that they get two tries. If they're unsuccessful and do a lot of digging, they must stop and find someone else to do the job—preferably someone with more skill or experience. Strike two, you're out.

Occasionally, I'll notice that when I tell them they must draw from my hand, their eyes fill with fear. They stumble around and can't figure out which tube goes with which test. These are the newbies. As rude as it sounds, I don't let newbies draw blood. I'm very unpopular when I announce I'd like them to go get their superior and have them do the draw. Some argue, but most sheepishly walk away and get their boss. The boss most often does a wonderful blood draw, even with the scowl on her face.

I realize just because someone's new doesn't automatically mean they won't be good at what they're doing. Nonetheless, I've had enough experience to know that it often does mean just that. I go with the odds. Often, I leave the lab or hear the door of my hospital room slamming shut and know I haven't made any friends. I'm sure all kinds of nasty things are said behind my back. When I look down at my hand, and see that my veins are still in one piece, I really don't care.

What I Know Now:

Remaining aware of what is being given to you and on what schedule can be taxing. Establishing boundaries with those caring for you can be very uncomfortable. Nonetheless, this is what must be done in order to ensure you're getting the best care. Don't lay back and relax. Keep an eye on what is being done to you and learn how to ask people to step back and change their approach. Trust me, you'll be happy you did.

Patterns of Illness

Journal entry from December, 2001:

I've found that the patterns of illness are hard to break. Although I'm mostly healthy now, I still react to my environment with many of the same thought patterns and emotional patterns I had when I was very sick. When I see a flight of stairs, I still react with dread, despite the fact they no longer pose an obstacle to me. When I see a full schedule on my calendar, I react with fear and panic, convinced I won't have the strength and energy to get through the day. This is simply not true.

There are certainly patterns that have diminished over time. I no longer fear household chores like laundry. Somewhere along the way, my body and mind have recognized that it no longer poses a threat to my well-being. That's why it still surprises me when I have a strong reaction to things like stairs and my schedule.

I try and talk to myself in a reassuring tone, saying there's nothing to worry about anymore. That helps for a moment, but the emotions are so deep they resurface at the next turn.

It makes me sad that my body and mind have been through so much difficulty that I react to the world in such a fearful way. I pray that, as the years pass with good health still in tact (God willing) these patterns will continue to dissipate and I will find a deeper healing for the wounds that have caused such emotion.

Those Who Know ...
Do What They Know

So, you've gotten the test results back and it looks like you have a health issue that needs to be addressed. It's a bit outside the scope of your general practitioner but you trust him/her enough to guide you on where to go next. Or, maybe you don't, and you go to someone recommended to you from elsewhere. Do you know that where you happen to land will most likely dictate your medical course of action?

Doctor Knows Best—But Which One?

My father has a history of clogged arteries in his heart. He's had two stents placed. Despite this history, it was still a shock when his general practitioner informed him he was developing a similar kind of blockage in his kidney's artery. While he was familiar with the workings of the human heart, dealing with kidney disease was well outside my father's knowledge base.

Like a responsible patient would, he sought the guidance of various experts. In the end, he was faced with a shocking list of possible treatments to ponder. These included various medicines, dialysis, kidney transplant and renal surgery.

The heart doctor was his first stop. My father trusted his opinion immensely; they had a history. This doctor insisted the best option was to load my dad down with various kinds of blood pressure medications. At one point he was taking so many he could barely stay awake.

When he sought the counsel of a nephrologist, the doctor who specializes in renal medicine, he got a completely different view of his treatment options. They spoke with him about kidney transplants and dialysis. They even wanted him to sit through a tutorial on the function, cost and resources for in-home dialysis machines. In addition, they were adamant that he not bother with the renal stent surgery option: the risks were too high and the success rate not very good. He left that office with his head spinning.

Upon the family's urging, he also visited with a top renal surgeon at the same hospital where I had my transplant. The surgeon strongly believed he was a good candidate for the renal surgery that would place a stent in the blocked renal artery. The surgeon thought, without a doubt, this was the best course of action for his problem. Among the reasons, he cited very high success rates and the ability to get off of many of the blood pressure medications post-op. In fact, he was astounded by the number of meds my father was taking, and urged him to narrow it down by at least half of the current dosages. His belief was that if the issues couldn't be managed on half of his current drug regimen, surgery was certainly the best option.

Three different doctors, experts in their fields, and three completely different ways to treat the same problem. My parents left each consultation more confused than when they arrived. One doctor seemed to indicate that my father was in serious renal failure while others indicated that he was only in the very early stages and had plenty of time to make decisions. Each one presented a strong case for why they felt it best to proceed as they advised, often at the same time discounting the treatment plans of the other practitioners. It was a very stressful time for my parents as they hacked their way through the information at hand and tried to make the best decision.

What I Know Now:

Medical doctors typically believe in using medicine before surgery. Surgeons usually see the answers to your problems in surgery. A specialist will see you through that specialty's filter. When you walk into any particular office, you're walking into a certain perspective and a certain philosophy.

For many medical issues, there's no concrete and universal treatment plan. Often, however, when you speak with a doctor who has a passion for what he does, it will be presented as if there's one clear choice. Although it may be overwhelming, it's important to shop around, gather up all of your options and decide for yourself which treatment plan makes the most sense to you. That may mean going with one doctor in particular or that may mean combining the expertise of more than one. As always, you're in the driver's seat.

No one would go through all the years of medical school and additional years to learn a specialty if they didn't believe in what they were doing. Know that when you're getting a doctor's opinion, they're representing their training and their passion. They may have the answer for you or they may not, despite their compelling views!

To a Very Special Doctor

A letter written shortly after I was told I had approximately six months left to live

Dear Doctor N,

I want you to know how honored and privileged I've felt being one of your patients over the last few years. You've always approached me as a human being and seem to have genuine interest in my life and my feelings. Your passion for the work you do is obvious, and your compassion for your patients is astounding. No matter what happens to me, I will always feel lucky to have known you.

When I saw you in clinic last week, I was very moved by your emotion. I deeply appreciate your sadness that my life is drawing to a close. I also appreciate you being upfront, answering my questions honestly. Although six months doesn't seem like a lot of time, it's still good to know that I have that time left to spend with my family, say goodbye to those I love, and tie up any loose ends.

While I find your compassion and concern marvelous, I wanted to share with you where we disagree. You apologized to me for not being able to find a cure for chronic rejection in time to save my life and all of the lives around us that are succumbing to it. There's no need for apologies or guilt. You've dedicated your life to saving your patients and you've done an extraordinary job in an extraordinary specialty.

It seems to me that you've also formed a belief along the way that death is a failure. I want you to know that, from where I stand, death is most certainly *not* a failure. *There are many forms of healing and death is merely one of them.* I hope that someday you'll be able to let that feeling go.

You and your team have enabled me to live years past what I would have without your intervention. I feel lucky to have stayed on earth a little longer and done all the things I've done … while taking deep breaths! When it's time for me and I've gone, please don't feel sad that you couldn't "fix" me. Please don't feel badly that you haven't done enough. Just know how much I appreciate all you've done and that I'm perfectly at peace with leaving here and going home. I like to think I'm simply graduating early!

Your sincere feelings are very appreciated. I only hope that the sadness you feel over losing many of your beloved patients doesn't discourage you from continuing the incredible work you do. You're truly one in a billion.

With great respect and love,

Tiffany

Alternative Medicine

I have not been shy about going outside of Western medicine to seek the possibility of relief. Many of the concepts presented in Eastern medicine make sense to me. In my mind, it would be silly to assume that our doctors have all the answers.

When I first began experimenting with different alternative treatments, around 1995, my doctors looked at me like I had six heads. Some were respectful, albeit not thrilled, about my exploration. Some were outspoken in their disbelief and practically laughed in my face.

I have seen attitudes change since then. Some doctors now actually recommend trying certain treatments while others just agree to disagree. There has been progress within the integrative medicine approach, but many still question its validity. Often the arguments surrounding alternative medicine revolve around whether or not it's the placebo effect. My question is: "How many pills that were prescribed by my Western doctor worked because of the placebo effect?" If it works, who cares?

The important question is how to find the right alternative practitioner and therapy that will work for your situation. As for whether or not to share your alternative medicine experiences with your Western doctor, that's up to you. It's always good to check in and make sure there aren't any clear contraindications. Just be aware, you may have to gear up and justify your decisions.

A Wonderful Compliment:

I was very sick when I discovered that chiropractic adjustments provided me with tremendous relief. I was only a year or so away from getting my first transplant and I, literally, spent hours coughing every day. This kind of coughing was deep and violent, and it began to affect even my skeletal structure. I developed a significant hunch and was unable to straighten up.

I began seeing my chiropractor, and, within weeks, I was standing straight. He helped readjust the way my bones had become accustomed to being, as well as stretch my stomach muscles so they were no longer pulling me down and forward. This allowed me to get more air into my lungs because there was simply more space in my torso. I felt taller and looked healthier. It's all really quite logical if you think about it! I was in less pain and found this therapy to be invaluable to my quality of life. It was soon after that I discovered the benefits of acupuncture as well.

Together, these two therapies helped me control my symptoms with no pain medications, and, I believe, slowed the progression of my disease. By helping me manage the symptoms—other than the infections—that contributed to my inability to breath, I had less to contend with and felt better than I would have without the alternative treatments. This meant fewer trips to the doctor, less medications and less hospitalizations. These alternative treatments were not wizardry, they were a wonderful complement to the care I was receiving at the CF clinic.

A Wolf in New Age Clothing:

He came highly recommended to me. He had been one of those people who almost defied physics in the magic he could perform to help the sick. A woman I had close connections with would see him once a week and spoke of all the amazing things he knew about her body and how to heal it; something the Western doctors had been able to do.

I made an appointment and was anxious to see what this man had to offer me and my ailing health. He lived far out in the country near a beautiful lake. The house was large and he had an entirely separate building as his office. I got the impression he made good money doing this healing work.

When I went inside, he was with another client. I sat in the waiting room and noted the many Native American tchotchkes around me. Someone who had been trained by Native American healers perhaps? I was excited to find out where his skills came from.

His client left and he came out to meet me. Although I was startled by his appearance, I wasn't surprised. He had long grey and white hair and so many crystals dangling from everywhere that I hardly noticed his weathered face. He spoke to me in a soft voice, in a tone I'd heard many times, one filled with pity and sympathy.

He took me back to his large "treatment area" that was reminiscent of a covered greenhouse. Strange art, presumably his, was sitting on the floor, leaning against the walls, encircling the room. We went to the very back corner where he had me sit in a chair and he sat at his desk.

He began by asking me to put both feet on the floor, close my eyes and breathe deeply. I had been studying various forms of meditation and was very familiar with this routine. I obliged with the exception of the breathing deeply part, as I was unable to do so at that point. I naturally began to go into my meditative state, a place I was comfortable with. He began talking to me about going inside myself and feeling the white light starting at my feet and moving up my legs into my torso, my arms, and my head.

While the meditation was routine, his comments were not. He was acting as though he could see the light inside me and made comments as though he could tell if I was successful or not in my mediation. It rang phony to me and I decided to test him. He proved to me he wasn't really seeing anything when he began dramatically oohing and ahhing at my internal progress when, in truth, I wasn't even following the meditation. This guy was beginning to look like a quack.

After the meditation was done, he stared at me, intensely, for what seemed like weeks. I was irritated with his charades and stared back. Eventually, he asked me in that liquid tone, "What do you think?"

I said "I'm just waiting."

He replied "No, what do you think of me?"

I answered, "Not much."

He was clearly upset and flustered by my lack of wonderment. He spoke to me in a condescending tone that put me on the defensive. He launched into a lecture about how I needed a spiritual tradition and that when I found one I would be much more centered. Translation: "I'm the guru here. You have no idea what you have in front of you and you should be swooning by now."

Little did this man know I did have a very strong spiritual tradition; one I'd dedicated much of my life to. His rude assumptions based on my appearance alienated me even further, but, for some naive reason, I still let him treat me. I guess I was still hoping for the miracle.

We moved to the table and he hooked me up to a machine that he had "adapted." I recognized the machine; they had the same one in my chiropractor's office. The wires looked the same but it didn't have the same sticky pads. Instead it looked more like small coat hangers at the ends. He bragged that this was the only machine of its kind.

He was miffed again when I told him my chiropractor had the same one, and he quickly replied, "But does hers measure your aura?"

No, hers didn't measure a person's aura because that would be silly! By definition, an aura changes, second to second, based on your emotions and the environmental stimuli. Even if he could measure it, what would be the value in that? Weary of our battle of spiritual wills, I agreed he had the only one and shut up. I was losing hope and was ready to go home.

It would be a long time before I could leave this man's lair. I was on his table for two hours, getting my "aura checked by the only machine of its kind." Finally, it was time to go and he was going to make up some homeopathic remedies. I declined. Again, he was flustered, but offered a big discount because I didn't want his remedies. He charged me $300.00! This was a discount; he normally charged at least $500.00 a session. I threw my check at him and got out of there as fast as I could. I obviously never went back.

I shudder to think what might have happened to my bank account if I hadn't had the presence of mind to question this man's abilities. I like to think I wouldn't have fallen under his spell like my friend did, but someone who promises health in the face of death can be quite an alluring thing. These are the kinds of alternative "practitioners" that give all the good ones a bad name.

He promised me the things I most wanted, health and happiness, and used those things to lure me into his practice, despite his limited ability to deliver the goods. As for my friend, he became her primary source of treatment and strongly advised her not to seek counsel outside of his techniques. The result was that she went into early kidney failure and he tried to treat it with his remedies but she became so ill she had to "defy" him and seek out a Western doctor. She realized he would have let her die before relinquishing control of her health. This is when she chose to stop seeing him.

What I Know Now:

Any good practitioner will be open to anything that will help you, and will never put your life in jeopardy to support his or her own agenda.

For symptom control, alternative medicine can be very helpful. Often, my underlying disease was being treated by Western medicine, but things like nausea and back pain were not. I find it a much more appealing choice to get acupuncture for those symptoms rather than add more pills to my regimen that have their own side effects.

I'm wary of alternative medicine practitioners who boast they can cure anything. I'm wary of alternative medicine practitioners who deny the value of Western medicine. I'm wary of alternative medicine practitioners who want to be your exclusive source for health care.

Patients must make sure that they are being safe in the alternative therapies they choose. For example, immune suppressed people should not take herbs to help with colds or other problems. I knew a transplant patient who didn't realize how the herbs worked, they boosted his immune system and he went into rejection. Alternative practitioners may not always understand the nuances of your disease and treatments so that needs to be your responsibility.

Other than those warnings, I'm very grateful for the practitioners who have cared for the parts of me that were being neglected by Western medicine. I've tried conventional alternative medicine (i.e. acupuncture and chiropractic) as well as the more "out-there" therapies like plant spirit medicine and shamanic journeying. Many of them I found benefited me emotionally, spiritually and/or physically. There were a few I found to be harmful.

Because the field of alternative medicine is still considered a fringe endeavor, it is not as regulated as conventional medicine. Because of this, it's difficult to know what you'll find when you walk into any given office. It can be difficult to find the balance between being open-minded and cautiously aware, but I believe that's the balance that must be found.

In Health Care, Everyone Counts

When thinking about health care, most people usually think about doctors first and nurses second. While they're certainly the main players, that doesn't mean other people in the medical arena can't have a major impact.

Does a Dangerous Tongue Always Come with the Sponge Bath?

A good friend of mine woke up in the middle of the night to find herself paralyzed on the left side of her body. She somehow pulled herself over to the phone and called someone to come get her and take her to the hospital.

She was admitted, of course, and began her long journey back to health with test after test. As it turned out, she had a form of a stroke called vasculitis. She was terrified so I spent the night in the chair next to her as often as I could.

One morning, only a few days after she had fallen so ill, a young nursing assistant came in to give her a sponge bath. My friend, weak and scared, was made to feel even more vulnerable by the stripping off of her clothes. As the woman washed her they began to talk. My friend told her what had happened and why she was partially paralyzed.

The nursing assistant began to ask her about Jesus, and I didn't think much of it since my friend is a devout Christian. Soon the conversation slid into why this had happened to her, and the nursing assistant offered her opinion that it was due to her sinning nature. She surmised that if my friend hadn't been such a sinner this wouldn't have happened.

As a little back-story on my friend, she was very kind and very innocent. She'd never been married, never been intimate and loved to teach children. Also, as I mentioned, she was a devout Christian.

To my surprise my friend didn't defend herself. Naked and shivering, she began to cry and accepted the theory presented by the nursing assistant. I was enraged and told the woman to leave immediately.

In my friend's state it took me hours to help her see that the words spoken were cruel and untrue. After that day, I was never sure my friend completely believed that her ailment wasn't caused by her sinning.

Just a nursing assistant? Yes, with a dangerous tongue and too much access to patients. I'm proud to say I got her fired.

Flailing and Mopping:

After my first transplant I was in ICU for a week. I was intubated and on lots of pain medications. Every morning I would be woken up by the cleaning lady asking me if I was okay. I was baffled! Why did this woman keep waking me from my peaceful sleep?

One morning I was dreaming that I was cleaning out my closet (riveting, I know). I woke up slowly and saw that I had my arms out stretched and was acting out the dream with my hands. It dawned on me that this must be why the cleaning lady would wake me up! My morphine dreams were so real I had been acting them out and it would appear I was in distress.

I wish I could tell that woman how much I appreciate her concern and how comforting it is to know she looks out for people in the hospital. It's so nice to know that some people just care about patients, no matter what the job description.

What I Know Now:

In health care, never underestimate the power of one person's role. Never fail to report a callous care giver or employee because chances are, it's not an isolated incident. Always thank people for their kindness. It's a beautiful gift.

A Letter to the Overwhelmed Med Student on the Pulmonary Floor

This letter was written during one of my many in-patient experiences and could have been written many times, to many different students!

My Dearest Med Student,

I see the look of fear in your eyes when you come into my room. It warms my heart to meet you before you've decided that you know oceans more than me. Your sweetness makes me want to help you.

I've been on this ride for a very long time. I've lived with all stages of illness. I know my disease process and my options. I've learned how to be an effective self-advocate. I tell you these things not to brag. It's to confess that despite my ability to care for myself, at the end of the day, you and I have to work together, and you still hold a lot of power.

I used to think a lot of doctors were stupid. I used to think a lot of doctors were cruel. I don't think that as much anymore. I think you've taken on something that's beyond your expectations. I think the job you do is difficult beyond your wildest dreams.

Those of you who work in the medical field face quite a predicament. Taking care of the sick and the dying is a job. A job is something you do to make money and then go home. At the same time, that "job" has an impact on people that could alter the very course of their lives.

I don't envy the kind of emotional and mental balancing act it must take to work in this field. It's my opinion, however, that doing this job well means more than knowing which medications interact with other medications or how many CCs go into that syringe.

There will be a time when you come to a crossroads. You'll have gained enough knowledge to make you feel confident. You'll have dealt with enough difficult patients to make you feel annoyed and maybe a little self-righteous. You'll have a choice: you can become one of the doctors who stops listening to those they treat or you can remain one of the ones who do listen. You can disconnect from what you're doing and see the lives before you as cases, or remember they're mothers, grandfathers, children. You can go to work to medicate people or you can help them heal. These are very different choices.

In my life, I've had doctors who inspired me to fight to live longer. Likewise, I've had doctors who made me want to give up. The influence you hold is powerful and beyond your imagination. You call this your job, but, really, isn't it so much more? We have much to teach each other, you and I.

Being a doctor is an awesome responsibility. It's my experience that the good ones are never so bold as to think they're up to the task.

~The Difficult Patient in Room 6543

The Power of Expectation

I heard about an experiment once where they blindfolded people and put different kinds of tastes in their mouth: salty, sweet, sour. The first time they told them what to expect before they placed it on the tongue, and, no matter how bitter or distasteful, the reactions were minimal. Then they started giving them false information, like telling them it was going to be salty and it was really sweet. Despite the fact that what they got might have actually been more pleasant to taste, the reactions were strong and they were mostly anger or frustration.

I think of this experiment often. As a patient, it can be extremely upsetting to have a result you hadn't anticipated. Aligning your expectations with what's likely to occur is essential.

Forewarned = Forearmed:

When I sat down with my surgeon, he told me that, after the lung transplant, I was going to feel like I "got hit by a Mack truck." I was startled by his candor, but his strong warning allowed me to brace myself for what lay ahead.

After my transplant surgery, I *did* feel like I'd been hit by a Mack truck. Since I was expecting it, however, I wasn't worried and was much better equipped to cope with the pain. I knew what I was experiencing was normal and I was able to almost relax into the discomfort.

When I sat down with my GI doctor before a G-tube placement—which is a day procedure—he told me it would feel like I "got stung by a bee." It didn't feel like a bee sting; it was very painful. For weeks every twist of my torso, every jolt of my step sent shock waves from my stomach throughout my body. I spent my time worrying and crying. This was supposed to feel like a bee sting, right?

I naturally assumed that because my experience was so vastly different than what I'd been told, something must be terribly wrong. In fact, there wasn't anything unusual about my pain except the lack of warning. I'd been misled by my doctor.

When I think back on both experiences, the trauma of my G-tube was much more intense. I remember telling people I'd rather have a transplant than a g-tube placement! Wow. The power of expectation.

Expect Not, Dear Guinea Pig!:

Three years after my second transplant, research started coming out that showed a connection between chronic rejection—a recipient's greatest enemy—and acid reflux. The theory being that if we have high PH acid in our stomach, we can aspirate that acid in our sleep. This, in turn, causes damage to the airways and may trigger chronic rejection.

The solution for this is a surgery called a Nissen fundoplication. It's essentially a way to wrap part of the stomach around the esophagus so that acid can't reflux into the airway. Because of my history, my team strongly urged me to have this surgery.

I wasn't having any problems with my lungs and I resisted for many months; the idea of undergoing another surgery was quite unappealing. Deciding whether or not to go ahead with an elective surgery, that would help me only in theory and when I was in a stable, healthy condition, was a very difficult decision. Ultimately, I chose to move forward in the name of "doing everything I can to preserve my health."

There was just one problem. Despite insisting I speak with another patient with my body size—I'm small and have trouble keeping weight on—as well as my history of transplant, nobody was able to produce such a person. All the cases presented to me were men. In addition, tests indicated I needed to have a second procedure called a pyloroplasty. This would be the solution to problems that were likely to occur as a result of the first procedure! Again, nobody I talked to knew anybody who'd done both of these surgeries at the same time. I was going into uncharted waters.

You'd think that going into the surgery so blind, I'd have no real expectations. It didn't work that way. I still sought out people to give me some sense of what was to come. I spoke with a nutritionist about my concerns regarding losing weight. She gave me a liquid diet that would allow me to take in 2,500 calories a day so I could keep my weight on, even when I wasn't able to eat solid foods. Piece of cake! My surgeons told me I'd be able to go back to work in ten days. Easy as pie! My transplant team told me I'd feel badly for a day or so and then I'd be fine. Walk in the park!

As you might have guessed, it wasn't a piece of cake, easy as pie or a walk in the park. I was unable to ingest *anything* for over a week. I was so severely nauseous they had to use every drug possible to keep me from retching and tearing the internal sutures. (I still had a few horrible bouts of retching anyway.) I lost over ten pounds and I was only 109 to begin with. For weeks I was absolutely miserable and completely unprepared.

My reaction was anger and regret. I was angry at myself for doing the surgery. I was angry at the nutritionist who acted as though she had a lot of experience with this procedure. I could barely drink half a glass of water, much less 2,500 calories a day! I was angry with all of my doctors who didn't tell me how hard this was going to be. I deeply regretted my decision.

It wasn't until I healed, a month or so later, that I was able to take a step back and see what had been so obvious all along. This hadn't been done before so why would I expect anyone to be able to predict the results? I was looking for answers and was only receiving guesses. To my credit, the guesses were really presented as facts.

I sometimes wonder if I'd have gone through with it if I'd gotten the honest answer: "We just don't know." Sometimes, when you're facing something scary, you want reassurance so badly that the truth doesn't seem clear. I ignored the facts and listened with my fear.

If I had to do it over again, under the exact same circumstances, I'd resist the urge to find "answers" and look at it as an exploration. I'd assume the worst. My only expectation would be that I was going to be the person that taught them how to do it better next time.

As it turned out, a friend of mine had the same surgery a few months after mine. They had already made some major adjustments to how things were done and her road was smoother than mine. I like to think my suffering helped other patients suffer less.

What I Know Now:

Of course, you can never know exactly what the future holds. Sometimes, things go wrong and your experience is much worse than the normal case. Sometimes, what's horrible for one person is a breeze for another. Sometimes, there's no normal and you have to decide if you're willing to be a pioneer. No matter what, there's always going to be the variable that's the individual.

Having said that, a patient's most powerful coping mechanism is often properly-aligned expectations. This includes pain levels, surgical recovery times, medication side effects, length of stay in the hospital—the list goes on and on. Talk to your doctor and ask the scary questions about best and worst case scenarios. Seek out fellow patients with similar medical histories who've had the treatment before you. If no precedent's been established, assume there will be difficulty. It's much better to prepare for the worst and hope for the best than to prepare for the best and be surprised by the worst.

There's a Limit

A patient is often stereotyped based on a diagnosis or medical history. People may assume that, because I'm a frequent flyer, that simple things like blood draws are a breeze for me. I was surprised to learn that it's common for the opposite to be true.

A Lower Tolerance for Pain:

I was in the hospital suffering from the effects of a tick bite and had been diagnosed with Rocky Mountain Spotted Fever. I wasn't feeling very well, as you might imagine, and was getting much needed rest. It was two in the morning and I was sound asleep.

A phlebotomist came into my room and startled me by turning on the bright lights over my head. I tried to keep my eyes closed and not let the rumblings of her cart and the scrunching of her papers wake me up so much that I couldn't fall back asleep. Before I knew what was happening, she'd put a needle in the bend of my elbow. I didn't have the chance to tell her I preferred to be poked in my hand so I hoped for a viable vein in my arm.

Still working to keep myself quiet enough to be able to fall back to sleep, I tried to remain calm while she dug around for a vein. Eventually, I was relieved to see she had succeeded in getting some blood. When she left, however, I was met with an excruciating pain in my arm. I can only assume she managed to hit a nerve because the pain was nearly unbearable. I didn't bother to call the nurse; I figured there wasn't anything they could do for this problem. Instead, I cried for hours, trying to let myself accept the pain and just go back to dreaming. I was unable to sleep again until about six o'clock when the pain finally started to diminish.

An hour later, the intern came in to wake me up and start my morning of questions and more tests. I'd lost hours of sleep due to pain, but there was no sympathy on the part of the staff. I truly don't think they understood how a blood draw could hurt so much. I wouldn't have understood either if it hadn't happened to me.

Had it not been for the hundreds of prior blood draws and IV catheters that had made my veins so fragile, I doubt this would have happened. My body had reached a physical limit as to how much poking and prodding it could stand.

The accumulation of years and years of invading my veins had make simple blood draws a painful event even under the best of circumstances. It has gotten to the point that I often cry all the way home after a routine blood draw. This kind of accumulation isn't something people in the medical field seem to be aware of.

Cell Memory:

I never thought much about cell memory until I experienced its effects. When it came to surgery, I'd always had the attitude that I was asleep, so what they did under anesthesia didn't matter much. In fact, I was never concerned about the transplant surgery itself because I got to sleep through it. I was always more worried about the recovery period after. While that's a partially true statement, I've found that it's a bit naïve.

One day, when I was playing a game, I found myself in a very similar physical position to the position I was in when I had both of my surgeries. I was laying still and my arms were immobile above my head. I almost immediately began to feel an emotional discomfort. I tried to ignore it so I could stay in the game but the feelings grew. Soon, I was feeling strong anxiety and began to cry. I left the game and went off on my own.

What happened next was a confusing series of emotions. I began to sob uncontrollably. I still had no idea what was happening to me and why I was so upset. Somebody came over to me and asked what was wrong. I had no logical explanation for my emotional outburst. The only thing that was coming to my mind was the word "violation" and an intense feeling to match it. I finally put the pieces together and realized that my body was speaking to me and my feelings weren't coming from an emotional place, but a physical one.

It was almost as if I could remember being in the transplant position for seven hours; my hands locked above my head and my ankles strapped down. There was a part of me somewhere that remembered the discomfort of this and how desperately I had wanted to move away from the hands and tools invading my insides. I sobbed for a solid hour and let my cells release the pain of my two surgeries. "I" had been asleep, but clearly there was a part of me that wasn't.

After my second transplant I was facing another surgery on my stomach. This was a laparoscopic procedure and, by all accounts, a "minor surgery." My reaction to the idea, however, wasn't minor in any way. I was terrified of the thought of it and fought the team tooth and nail about having it done.

It finally occurred to me that part of my reaction wasn't coming from my conscious self, but rather my cells once again speaking to the pain of their violation. Certainly, this laparoscopic procedure would be far less of a "violation" but my body objected just the same. Again, I could feel fear and resistance to being cut and invaded by medical tools.

I went forward with the surgery, but was aware that there was a part of me that needed nurturing and assurance, and it wasn't my mind. My body has a voice. I just have to learn how to hear what it needs to say.

What I Know Now:

My body's been through so much cutting, poking and prodding that it's reached a certain limit. I now try to communicate this to my caregivers before a procedure because I know their expectations of me may be inaccurate. They think because of all that I've been through that I must be an "old pro" and therefore will be unflinching in the face of medical procedures. Not so!

I've found, in talking with other patients, my experience is not unique. Having a wealth of accumulated medical experiences can results in a change in how the body and mind react to pokes and prods. When you've been around the block, you might start noticing disproportionate reactions to medical stimuli. Be kind to yourself and your body. Factor your body's silent feelings into the formula that comes with undergoing any procedure, large or small.

Truthfully Yours

A letter written when I was dying of chronic rejection

Dear Dr. Batistte,

I heard you talking about me in clinic today. You forgot to shut the door all the way. I wasn't very surprised by what I heard. I could tell by the look in your eyes that you didn't like coming into my room. I guess I thought you just didn't like your job, but now I know you just don't like me. I wish that didn't bother me, but it does.

Do you understand that what you see when you enter my exam room is merely a snapshot of my life? Sure, you see a frail girl on oxygen who's angry and bitter. Do you think that's who I am? I suppose you do. What else would you think of me since that's all you know?

I *am* angry and bitter. I'm angry that I'm dying and yet I still have to come to clinic every month. You've told me there's nothing you can do for me, so why do you make me haul my oxygen tank all the way from my home to the hospital? Is it so you can keep up with my statistics? Well, I stopped caring about my statistics months ago. I wish you'd just leave me alone and let me be in peace.

Instead, I follow your orders like a sheep and show up to clinic every month, tired and irritable. I heard you call me "difficult." I know you've written me off as a problem patient. I would guess you've even labeled me the crowd favorite: non-compliant. Is your perception that limited? Your compassion so shallow?

Perhaps I'm a problem patient. If you'd like to call me that, I won't dispute it. Where I have a problem is when that becomes the beginning and the end of my definition.

I'm a problem patient and I'm a survivor.
I'm fun and I'm too serious.
I'm compassionate and I'm judgmental.
I'm fulfilled and I'm empty.

I'm surrounded by loved ones and I'm lonely.
I'm everyone and I'm only myself.
I'm just like you and I'm nothing like you.

I'm sorry that I've made your work day a little harder, a little longer. I'm trying to live with terminal illness and you're trying to get to lunch. Our agendas are so different.

You've hurt me today with your overly simplistic label of my state of mind. The problem is, your label is seen as a scientific fact. I mean, it went in my chart, didn't it? That makes it real and concrete.

I heard you behind that crack in the door say there wasn't anything you could do for me. I heard you describe how difficult I am, which makes it impossible to work with me. I wish you knew how wrong you were.

We wanted different things from each other, you and me. You wanted a smile, perhaps? A warm welcome? I wanted understanding. Today, neither of us got what we wanted but it didn't have to be that way. I wish I'd never heard you behind that door.

I'm angry with you. I don't have much warmth in my heart for you. The only kind thing I can say today is that I hope you never have to face the same kind of one-dimensional assessment you've placed on me. There's little in this world that hurts me more than being so misunderstood.

Truthfully yours,
Tiffany

Truce

Everyone has their own coping mechanisms. Some people I've known use denial. They know as little as possible about their illness, their medications and their prognosis. From what I've observed, this manifests as chronic worry about every tingle and unusual sensation that could mean more illness. I've also seen denial manifest as a manic need to do, do, do—even when the body is too tired to continue. There's always another job to do and there's never a moment without noise.

Some people I know use self-pity. They see themselves as victims and rely on other people to "serve" them. Their identity is completely wound around being helpless and sick. This mentality continues even when the body is healed. From what I've observed, this manifests as a deep fear of failure and inability to embrace life.

I use positivism as my coping mechanism. I choose to see only the bright side of my illness and concentrate on all the lessons I've learned from being sick. I find a deep spiritual meaning in all that I've suffered and feel closer to God because of it. Sounds good right? If only it were that easy.

It took me nearly thirty-four years of living with severe illness to finally admit the other side of that story to myself, the side of the story that isn't so pretty. The truth is I disconnected from my physical self early in life. I found great comfort in viewing my body as merely a wrapper for my true self, the soul and mind that I call me.

That separation went beyond a metaphysical philosophy, however. At the darkest corners of myself I hated my body. I hated it to the extent that I wished it pain and suffering. I secretly believed it deserved every needle poke, every IV and every cut of the scalpel. I hated it so much that I blamed it for my life's struggles and felt that it had betrayed me by being genetically flawed. I was living within an entire belief system that was unknown to my conscious mind.

When I discovered this unconscious set of beliefs, I was terrified. This went against all that I thought I was and all that I thought I believed about my illness. I wasn't nearly as evolved as I liked to think I was!

As strange as it sounds, my body and I needed to have a conversation. My body was resentful that it had been violated with all the thousands of medical interventions, and I was resentful that my life had been interrupted over and over by a mutated gene. It was an internal conversation between three parts of myself: logic, the part I consider me and my physical self.

Logic told us life would be much better if we could learn to work together and be in harmony. Me and my physical self didn't even know how to take the first step toward putting the past sufferings behind us and come together as one.

As I write this, my body and I are in the early stages of figuring out how to be a team. We've called a truce and will work to have compassion for each other. I see that if I love my body more I'll treat it better. Perhaps I will *want* to eat well and exercise! (Maybe not) At the very least, I'll stop seeing it as a separate part of myself that's an enemy and recognize it as another part of what makes me who I am.

My body is an innocent in this scenario, just as I am. I see that now, and I'm working on forgiving a wrong that was never committed. I'm working on loving myself from every angle.

Pieces of Pain

It's my understanding, as a lay person, that pain is the tool the body uses to tell the brain that there's a malfunction happening somewhere in the body—like the engine failure light in a car.

It took me awhile to figure out that acute pain doesn't always indicate a disaster that requires you to pull over and get a tow truck. Likewise, chronic pain isn't always something that you can push through and keep on driving to the next exit. Pain can be confusing and that's why it should be approached consciously.

Heart Attack or Big Dinner?

When experiencing unexpected pain, often, the fear of what *may* be happening is equal to the physical sensation. This only causes the pain to escalate.

One weekend, a man I was dating declared he needed me to drive him to the emergency room. He was sure he was having a heart attack and was doubled over in pain. Scared, we rushed to the nearest hospital and he underwent a battery of tests. It turned out he had very bad gas.

After he mentally understood what was happening to his body and that he'd be okay, it was easy to get his fear and, by extension, his pain under control. The pain hadn't changed, only his understanding of it, but that was enough to greatly diminish his discomfort. After that, all he had to do was get over the embarrassment!

Let Me Let it Out:

I'll never forget the morning after my first transplant. I had barely slept a wink—machines had been beeping and nurses had been bustling all night long. The first visitor to my bedside was the mobile X-ray man. Normally, in order to get the chest X-ray, I would be rolled slightly onto my side and the film would slide behind me. Not this time. With no warning the X-ray man

47

began to shove the block of film under my back with surprising force. It was unbelievably painful but I was intubated and could not cry out for him to stop. He did this about four more times before he left.

I was still wincing from the X-ray experience when the physical therapists came in. Their job was to pound on my torso with cupped hands in hope that they might loosen any unwanted phlegm lurking in my new lungs. Normally, this is annoying but not at all painful. Not this time. Fresh from surgery, their pounding was like a jackhammer on my chest and I could barely stand it. I hit my morphine as much as possible and prayed for their speedy departure. Eventually, my prayers were answered and they left me. I held onto my sides, hopeful that the throbbing would soon stop.

My alone-time didn't last long. The second group of physical therapists arrived with shining faces. "Time for your walk!" they happily exclaimed. I had a transplant yesterday, my morning had been horrible and now it was time for *walking*? I could no longer hold back my tears.

Crying while intubated isn't pretty. I scared off the physical therapists and they ran to fetch my transplant coordinator. She came in quickly after they had gone. Her job was to calm me down. I tried to explain with hand gestures and nods, but, clearly, my point was not getting across. I just needed a break. That's all I wanted but, somehow, what I got was countless pep talks.

Since when is crying under those circumstances something to fix? Who wouldn't be crying after that kind of morning? I see it in so many places and in so many ways: tears in the hospital are strongly discouraged.

What's ironic is that releasing emotions decreases physical discomfort. A patient benefits on all levels as they begin to separate their emotional and physical pain. Once my emotions were tended to there was more strength left over to heal the body. After my cry, I was able to get up and take that walk.

I just needed to let it out. This all sounds quite logical but, I assure you, isn't a common practice in ICU.

Why Pain?:

A common example of an underlying belief system related to pain is: "Why is God allowing this to happen to me? I must be being punished."

Another common one is: "Why me? This isn't fair!"

My personal belief system was at one time: "I'm too *young* to be so sick. I shouldn't have to deal with sickness and death yet!"

Believing that you're being punished or that you somehow got a raw deal is going to breed feelings of anger, resentment, self-pity, and maybe even shame.

These kinds of belief systems are not helpful and don't do much in the way of lessening suffering. The trick is finding a new belief system, one that comes from your heart, not your head.

Sometimes I outgrow my belief system and it doesn't inspire me anymore. That's when I find a new one. I've replaced mine more than a few times over the years. My core belief system now is: "There's purpose in my suffering as I've learned much and can give much."

What I Know Now:

When I think of chronic pain, I think of depression and when I think of acute pain, I think of fear. Pain may make you depressed or question your purpose on earth. Pain may make you irritable or plain angry. None of these reactions are unusual or wrong, however, it's ideal if you can seek ways to cope with your pain that will enable you to see daylight at the moment the clouds part—even for a second.

There are medical ways to address pain and personal ways to address pain. It's important to think about which aspects of pain are within your control and which are not.

The Nuances of Pain
Medication and Addiction

When I was in my early twenties I was dating someone whose brother got into a terrible car accident. He was hit head on by a drunk driver. Among many injuries, his legs were shattered. He was, as you may imagine, in great pain. They had him on a morphine drip with a button he could push for an extra dose of pain medication. Despite the fact his pain wasn't always covered, he refused to press the button. He held a strong belief that if he took too much pain medication he'd end up addicted. He felt it was better to suffer the pain of his injuries rather than going through the difficulties of a narcotic addiction later.

In my life, I've witnessed varying degrees of this same idea, resulting in a strong resistance to taking much needed pain medication. I've also seen the opposite occur: a festive enthusiasm about the opportunity to take narcotics which resulted in an addiction. I've seen both sides of this coin in my own experience and have concluded that this kind of drug therapy must be approached with consciousness.

Save the Heroism and Take the Pill:

A few weeks after my first transplant, I was on a schedule of a common narcotic every four to five hours. One day, I was feeling very good. The nurse came in to give me my next pain med and I refused it, telling her I was fine and didn't need it at that time. About one hour later, I began to feel some discomfort. I called the nurse and asked for the pill. Quickly thereafter, an intense amount of pain set in.

She brought it to me and I eagerly swallowed it, waiting for relief. I grimaced and waited. I cried and waited. Nothing. I called the nurse again and told her I needed more pain medication. She explained that I would need special permission from the doctor and she'd give me more as soon as she heard from him. I waited another forty-five minutes before I got another dose. By the time she got to me, I thought I'd go mad.

What I learned that day was something I'd never known: if you let your pain get away from you, it will take a much larger dose to bring it back down to a comfortable level. I was trying to show off or be some kind of hero, and I learned my lesson. Falling behind on your pain medication can have disturbing results.

Pain or Puny?:

A week or so after my G-tube placement I was still on a narcotic for pain. While the site didn't hurt too badly, I kept taking my pain meds. At about two weeks, I was still reaching for my medication when I felt the familiar discomfort returning.

One day, as I was about to pop the pill in my mouth, I realized something. The symptoms that were causing me to reach for the bottle were no longer related to my surgery. They were the lethargy and icky feelings that show up when you're coming down off of the cloud of narcotic tranquility. It was almost like the early stages of having the flu.

Once I realized this, it became crystal clear to me how people become so easily addicted to these medications. If you aren't paying attention, it would be so easy to keep taking the narcotic to medicate the effects of not taking the narcotic.

I took notice that day, didn't take any more pills, and went through a day of feeling puny. I never felt the need for another pill after that. Now, I'm sure to evaluate if I'm taking a pain medication for the pain or for the more subtle side effects of the medication.

Good Intentions and Lots of Pills :

Doctors don't want their patients to be in pain. Pain management has become a key piece to practicing good medicine. My doctors had all the right intentions when they sent me home after my second transplant with three months worth of narcotic pain medication. I never took one pill after I left the hospital. I simply didn't have that much pain. Just because your doctor sends you home with it, doesn't mean you need to use it.

What I Know Now:

Dealing with pain and pain medication can be tricky. There's a balance that must be struck between not stopping too early and getting into trouble and continuing too long and getting into a different kind of trouble. The only answer can come from within.

It's the patient's job to do an internal survey and ask yourself where the pain is coming from and how severe it is. Those on the outside can only estimate your needs for pain treatment based on other people's experiences.

It's your job and responsibility to make the decision about that next pill based on your realistic view of your personal situation.

The Things We
Do to Sick People

Journal entry from May, 2006

Well, just when I thought I'd done it all, I got sick this week with something I'd never experienced. I had a really high fever, my joints ached so bad I could barely walk and I felt generally crappy. I went to the ER and, of course, they admitted me. The usual "We don't know what you have but we'll treat it with IV antibiotics" began. I was hoping they'd figure it out quickly because I have my big fundraiser coming up and have no time to spare. No such luck.

When the resident came in and told me I was scheduled for a PIC line placement, I had my normal reaction: tears and trembling. I fought the decision but with no success. Soon, I was being wheeled down to my least favorite place in the entire hospital: vascular radiology. They put my gurney up against the wall and I sat there like a bag of discarded garbage for what seemed like hours. No one spoke to me, no one even seemed to know I was there.

Despite my efforts to tune it out, I couldn't help but hear the conversations of the many doctors and nurses lollygagging in the hall. Most of what they had to say revolved around annoying patients and how cool they were for being doctors. It was a level of stereotypical doctor machismo that became almost comical. If it hadn't been for the fact that these were the people about to thread a mile long catheter through my arm and up to my heart, I might have laughed.

At one point, my IV machine started beeping, but it was ignored by everyone who passed by. I looked down to see there was a golf ball-size lump under my skin: my IV had infiltrated. It really started to hurt. I began to call out for someone to turn it off, but, still, I was invisible. I literally had to reach out and grab someone to get their attention. They shut off my IV and eons later wheeled me into the room that makes me cry.

It freaked everybody out that I was crying before I even got on the table. They didn't understand what the big deal was and I had learned long ago it was pointless to try and explain. I got on the table and they began to prep me for the procedure. I had a plastic sheet covering most of my upper body, including my face. It was quite claustrophobic. They strapped my arm down to a board at a strange and uncomfortable angle. They began to wipe me down with very cold Betadine. It was everywhere. The cold combined with my fever sent me into a shiver-frenzy. I was miserable.

It was at that moment it dawned on me: this would be terribly uncomfortable if I wasn't sick and scared to death. Add to it all of my maladies and it was downright awful. At that point, a phrase began to repeat in my head; "The things we do to sick people." It really is astounding what we make a person go through at their time of greatest dis-ease.

In the end, I was diagnosed with Rocky Mountain Spotted Fever. The treatment? *Oral* antibiotics. The PIC line stayed in a total of about one day and then we pulled it out. I doubt anyone besides me thought much of the needless pain and torture. The things we do to sick people!

System Failure

A letter written after the second transplant, while I was being reviewed by Social Security

To Whom It May Concern (And Who Does It Concern?):

For the most part, my political days are over. I marched on Washington a few times in the name of animal rights back in 1990–1991. Since then, most of my views have fallen more into the gray area. Even on those topics that I still get fired up over, I've lost faith that my lone opinion would have any influence on our massive governmental machine. When I'm caught in the crossfire of a political debate, for the most part I keep my mouth shut. I just don't see the point in arguing.

I'm writing a book that holds the potential to explore many of our country's political health care issues. In fact, sometimes I feel guilty for not being more involved in that aspect of patient care. Nonetheless, my focus tends to be more on my immediate experience and those things I deem to be within my power to affect as an individual. I don't really want to deal with politics.

That said, I'm feeling nervous about my future and I can't deny the impact our government could have on my life in the coming years. I began working a part time job about six months ago. Because I've been on disability and Medicare, it was my duty to report that I'd gone back to work. I'm not nervous because I've done anything wrong. I'm nervous because there are a lot of rules and I don't want to make any mistakes. If I do, I could potentially lose my disability status.

When people learn I'm on disability, they sometimes react with surprise. They think because I can walk, talk and stand upright that I should no longer be taking anything from the government. People may judge me because I'm on disability but what they don't understand is that I don't have the energy to work a full time job and I need Medicare. Medicare is directly linked to disability status.

I quit college because of my health, and therefore my skill set is limited to lower-paying jobs. I don't get benefits where I currently work, and even if I did, it's highly unlikely the office could handle someone like me on their group insurance. I have to approach my work schedule carefully so I can keep my disability status. If I lose my disability, I will begin to slide down the slope to the place where I lose my insurance. Can you even imagine the pre-existing conditions list on my private insurance application?

The chance that I could find work at a company that could provide me with insurance is slim. The possibility that I could pay for my own is simply impossible. What would someone like me do without insurance to pay for all of the transplant medications? The answer to that question is easy: they would die.

All of those ponderings are head-spinning but that doesn't even take into account what would happen if I became terminal or chronically ill for the third time. I'd have to quit my job and apply for disability again. What would happen to me in the meantime? How would I survive while I was waiting for Medicare to kick back in? The thought scares me to the bone.

It seems, I, and those like me, are between a rock and a hard place. If I work, I run the risk of losing necessary, life-sustaining government funded coverage. If I don't work I'm not fulfilling the entire goal of transplant: to live a more normal life. Like so many governmental programs, this is one more example of a good idea with no plan to help transition people from one end to the other.

I really have no right to complain. Compared to many other people, I've had it good. I've been able to be on Medicare for ten years and I've been able to have my father's insurance as back-up. Medicare paid for two very expensive lung transplants. My insurance pays for a regimen of medication that, in one month, costs about as much as my rent for a year. I'm very lucky to be alive and to have gotten the care my insurance provides. I really have no right to complain, but I'm going to anyway.

I didn't get this transplant so that I could sit at home on the couch and collect government money. I also didn't go through all of the pain and suffering so that I could live a more normal life, get a job and turn around and lose my insurance. How silly would it be, after all of this, to die because I couldn't afford to buy my transplant medications!

Things just don't add up. Medicare will pay for surgeries that cost a million dollars but won't follow through and pay for the medications that keep you alive afterwards—unless you promise to make less that a certain amount each month. I don't understand. All I want to do is go from being sick to making a contribution to the world. The organizations that got me well are the same ones standing in my way.

We need a bridge for people like me. Where is the bridge?
Sincerely,
Just Another Patient

The All-Important
Written Word

Communication between patients and doctors isn't always perfect. Likewise, communication between medical professionals isn't always perfect—or even close. There's hope and it comes in the form of the written word.

Make a Sign, Make it So:

When a person has a Nissen fundoplication, it usually prevents them from being able to vomit ever again. Nausea is a common problem for me, especially when pain meds are involved. Thank God my surgeon had been around the block a few times and understood the power of notes.

It's my experience that nausea is often taken very lightly by doctors and nurses. I tell them I'm nauseous and they respond with an "Oh, that's too bad." Meanwhile, there are many drugs that can be used to treat nausea.

I suppose my surgeon had found that same thing to be true because he printed out a big note and posted it above my bed: Treat Nausea Aggressively.

Guess what? Those people caring for me responded to that note as if God himself were speaking to them. I have never had people work so hard to medicate my nausea effectively. I still had a lot of problems with anesthesia-related nausea but I shudder to think how bad it could have been if he hadn't taken the time to make that note.

Do Not Disturb:

For those needing in-patient care sleep is a rarity. Between the night nurses hollering to each other down the hall during the wee morning hours, the twenty-four-hour-a-day blood draws and the revolving door of random visitors—professional and non-professional—finding time for rest isn't easy.

That's where the note comes in. Posting a note on the door stating that you're sleeping and to not disturb you until a set time worked wonders for me. There's just something about signs that people respect, and they'll usually adhere to their message.

Not Again:

A chart is something that accompanies you wherever you go in the hospital or doctor's office. A chart is also something that's written in but rarely ever read. Doctors and nurses tend to avoid the chart and go straight to the horse's mouth. For those of us who hate to repeat ourselves, it can be annoying when you discover you're relaying the same history again and again, to many different people.

Writing notes is a great alternative to saying the same information to every new face who walks in the room. Things like your medication regimen and your list of symptoms are great to have written down, both as an in-patient and an out-patient. Instead of saying it over and over, hand over your lists, sit back and relax.

Don't Remember It, Write It:

It's always smart to bring a pen and paper with you whenever you're meeting with a doctor. Medical details can be overwhelming and, over time, difficult to remember. Having a written record of the changes, options or diagnoses discussed allows you to revisit key elements later, when you're less inundated with information.

Processing new, health-related material is a multi-layered process. You should not expect to digest that information during the initial doctor's visit. When the patient is unable to take on the note-taking responsibility, either for emotional or physiological reasons, it's imperative that someone else take diligent notes instead.

You don't always get a second chance to go over things with the doctor so make sure to take advantage of the time you do have. Ask questions, get clear on everything being discussed and keep a record so you can refresh your memory later. You may think you'll remember everything when you're in the moment of listening, but, chances are, you won't.

What I Know Now:

Writing notes is one major step in helping to promote good communication for you and your team. It's not rude or arrogant; it's good common sense. Having a written note means you can relax more and feel like you don't need to defend yourself even in your sleep.

It can prevent frustration for the patient—repeating yourself can become annoying. Keeping notes for yourself can empower you to thoroughly review your options, thereby making better decisions.

Pen and paper: a great patient ally.

The Unpredictable ER

Whether you have acute symptoms in need of immediate attention, want to have something checked out during non-clinic hours or have an exacerbation of a chronic illness, chances are you'll, at some point, land in the same place: the emergency room.

This is a place with so much activity, so many life stories converging, they've made many hit TV shows about it. While I've met very few George Clooneys during my visits, I can see why this is a perfect setting for a great drama—or comedy, for that matter. This is the place in the hospital where anything goes. Car accident victims, gunshot wounds and people having heart attacks are all brought here. So is Fannie Falls A Lot with her ninth sprained wrist, as well as Penelope Puker who has the flu. The list of characters goes on and on, and suffice it to say, it's usually a bit chaotic.

Two Worlds Combine:

It was Sunday afternoon and I'd felt sick since Friday night. If it weren't for the fever I'd have waited for Monday, but I don't have the luxury of taking any chances with my health. My only choice was to head for the ER. Before leaving my house, I was sure to call my doctors, tell them when I planned to arrive and had them call ahead with orders and/or medications. The attending wasn't available, so I requested to speak with the resident-in-charge. The hope was that this type of pre-planning would get the wheels spinning—and maybe some tests ordered—before I even got there. This was only a hope.

The first thing I encountered at the ER—besides the full parking lot—was the reception desk. I had to remind myself that an ER isn't first come, first served. The most severe problems are seen first. I used to be shy when I came in and would only list my symptoms as my reason for being seen. What I've learned is that it's important to give a more well-rounded view of my situation to the people up front. That will help them understand the level of urgency in the situation and may help me get seen sooner.

I don't mean to suggest that I lie or exaggerate. I simply list pertinent information that will alert them to my needs. For example, I'm sure to let them know that, in addition to my fever, I'm a transplant patient and am immune-suppressed. Because of this, they work to get me in a room so I won't have to be exposed to other people's illnesses in the waiting room.

Once I'm in the back, it's important for me to get the ER doctors to consult with my team. Most physicians are happy to do so, but, on this trip, the ER docs resented outside influences and wanted to steer the ship.

For someone with my kind of history, my medical care is too complicated for it not to be handled by a specialist. They were dragging their feet about contacting my doctors, so I was sure to do it myself and got them involved as soon as possible. I used the phone in the ER to call my transplant coordinator directly and let her know what was happening.

Eventually, we were all on the same page and I was able to get the benefit of a functioning ER, one that worked in cooperation with and understanding of my primary care doctors' treatment plan. Had I not been aggressive, however, there's no telling how many days I could have sat around in that scratchy gown!

Bad Girl Going Downhill:

Some of the nicest, most talented nurses I've ever known were ones I met in the emergency room. Unfortunately, there are always exceptions.

I came into the ER one summer with a high fever I hadn't been able to control. I knew I'd be admitted, but the team wanted me to be seen at the ER until a bed was available. During the routine twenty questions, I told my nurse I'd taken four Tylenol to try and bring down my fever. She was appalled. She scolded me and told me I'd have to wait a long time to get any more. I certainly understood why taking four Tylenol was bad for me and I allowed her to make me feel like I'd done something very wrong. I sat quietly while my fever returned with a vengeance.

The hospital was packed full, and a bed wouldn't be ready any time soon. I got to feeling very poorly and asked for someone to take my temperature. It was 101. I requested some Tylenol and my nurse came in with her hair on fire. She told me I'd have to wait for another six hours before I could have another one. She wrapped me in blankets and told me again how wrong I was to have taken so many Tylenol.

I felt very vulnerable and very scared. I knew that a fever could cause my lungs to go into rejection. I knew I shouldn't let my fever continue but I was too weak to fight the woman.

By the time they found me a bed, my fever was 103.9. My doctors didn't care if I'd swallowed a bottle of pills that day; the priority was to reduce my fever. The team was almost as upset with the nurse as I was. For my particular health issues, that kind of fever had the potential to cause devastating results.

I learned I should never again doubt what I know and let myself be guilted into something. The solution to that problem was easy but I was too timid to carry it through. I should have enlisted help from my family, had them page my doctors and inform them of what was happening. The ER nurse was uninformed on the delicate nature of my disease, she wouldn't listen to my reasoning, and I should have found a way to take care of myself despite that.

What I Know Now:

Emergency medicine has to be one of the most difficult specialties. It's a place where the nurses and doctors need to know a little about a lot of things. It's a place of great distress and trauma. It's a place where people go when they have nowhere else to be seen.

There have been times when I'm in and out of the ER quickly, with very few bumps in the road. There are times that I've spent *days* in the ER waiting for a bed in the hospital. I've had very positive experiences and very negative experiences. One fact remains: the ER is an essential piece of the medical system pie.

That said, for those of us with specific problems, it's the luck of the draw as to whether those caring for you in the ER will know enough about your needs to treat you correctly. This is a place to stand up and flex your patient advocacy muscles. You may be delighted to find a doctor or nurse who knows a great deal about your specific ailment or you may find that you'll be doing a lot of on-the-spot educating.

Bottom line: Come prepared knowing the system and be willing to make it work for you.

Earth is Hard

I went to the hospital today for a clinic visit. On my way through the front doors, I spotted a woman in the corner crying, being consoled by an older man, perhaps her father.

In the lobby I saw a child in a wheelchair who was unable to control his body and looked as though he most likely couldn't speak. Next to him stood, I assumed, his mother and she looked absolutely exhausted.

As I made my way to the escalator, I saw a young woman who seemed to be mentally handicapped, screaming and flailing her arms. People who I assumed were her family surrounded her, and, with embarrassed faces, tried to control her tantrum.

At the top of the escalator I heard a man moaning and glanced over to see him on a gurney in the middle of the hallway. He was hooked up to an IV, unattended, and he looked to be in pain.

Walking into the clinic, I passed by two women and overheard one say, "The next step is chemotherapy. After that, well, I just don't know."

This wasn't an unusual day, I've seen worse on plenty of occasions. I'll never forget the mother I saw talking on the pediatric unit's pay phone, sobbing and relaying the very recent death of her daughter. That one still haunts me many years later.

The sights and sounds of the hospital are difficult to digest if you're paying attention. It's possible to barrel through and not notice the lives around you, but I've made a conscious choice not to do that. I try to drink in the pain, the suffering and the stories that are all around when I walk through the halls of any hospital, in any city, in any state.

I'm not alone in my suffering. I'm not the one that suffers the most. There's no shortage of people in pain. There's one phrase that runs through my head every time I journey through those hallways: *Earth is hard*. There's no doubt about it.

Be Careful Who You Listen To

While I'm a big fan of talking to anyone you can get your hands on in order to get more information about your medical situation, that endorsement does come with a disclaimer.

One Piece of the Perspective Pie:

Before my first transplant, I had a nurse who worked the night shift on the pulmonary floor who I became friends with over time. When I was in-house, he'd visit my room when things were slow. Back then, I was a night owl and he almost always found me awake and ready for a good talk.

Trusting his experience as a nurse, I asked him the questions that were weighing on my mind so heavily. I was wrestling with the idea of transplant and felt as though I was looking into a deep abyss, trying to find some answers. I was at the beginning of my transplant journey and was at a complete loss.

His replies were startling, to say the least. When I asked him if he thought transplant was a good option, he almost became angry. He told me stories of those who had suffered terribly because of an unsuccessful transplant. He insisted transplants were rarely helpful and usually harmful. The bottom line was clearly that transplant was the gateway to a painful, horrible death.

I took his words to heart, playing and replaying the images in my mind of the stories he told. I didn't want to be one of those patients. I steeled myself to the idea of transplant and resolved that it wasn't a good choice.

It wasn't until I got to know this man a little better that I realized how biased and one-sided his opinion had been. He hadn't done any research into transplant success rates. He had never worked in the transplant clinic. His entire opinion was formed by the handful of transplant patients he served as a nurse on the pulmonary floor. He didn't see the ones who weren't sick and the ones who were out living healthy, active lives. All he knew of transplant was rejection, complications and pain. His perspective was entirely skewed.

Once I realized this, I was able to see his opinion as merely one slice of the transplant perspective pie. While what he had witnessed was real, it was far from the entire picture. I let go of the images he'd planted in my mind and allowed myself to understand them as a possibility—no use for complete denial—while setting off to find the other pieces of the perspective pie.

Fast Food Fiasco:

While waiting for the transplant, one requirement was attendance at a bi-weekly meeting for patients and families. They called it a support group but it was more like an educational opportunity. There was very little crying and leaning on each other emotionally. Usually there was a speaker and, when there wasn't, people who'd already had their transplant would talk about their experiences.

There was one girl in particular who had a lot to say. One girl and her mother, I should say. This duo had the gift for gab and would dominate the conversation on many occasions. She and her mother were that breed of patient and family that seemed to find their identity as a patient or the parent of a patient. I might go so far as to say they *enjoyed* illness on some level and delighted in being the experts.

This girl, Pam, had received a double lung transplant but was experiencing on-again, off-again rejection. She would be placed on the list for another transplant and then get well and go inactive on the list. Her journey certainly had many twists and turns.

Looking to the post-transplant folks for a window into the transplant experience, I often spoke with Pam and her mother about things they'd been through. One story sticks out in my mind. Pam had been intubated due to some problems with her lungs and spent a few days in ICU. When she got better, the doctors pulled out her breathing tube. Pam was hungry and requested dinner from McDonald's. Her mom obliged and Pam began to scarf down a hamburger, fries and a Diet Coke.

Pam noted something odd: the food didn't satiate her hunger. She didn't feel like she had eaten at all. According to Pam and her mother, it was soon discovered that, due to the breathing tube, Pam's esophagus wasn't properly functioning and her food wasn't going into her stomach at all. According to them, it was going into her lungs instead.

This story, and many of Pam's other stories, haunted me for months. Post-transplant was a mysterious world to me and all of these freakish things happening to Pam only made it more so.

Over time, I began to see that Pam and her mother were prone to exaggeration and enjoyed shocking people with their horror stories. To this day, I have no idea which part of Pam's experiences were real and which (if any) were fabricated.

One thing was surely clear, however. Listening to Pam's stories didn't help me and only served to unnerve me. I stopped engaging Pam and her mother at the support group and am happy to report that I've never had a problem with any hamburger or fries ending up in my lungs.

What I Know Now:

I'm not a naturally skeptical person. When someone tells me something, I'll believe it long before I'd consider doubting it. Others may fall on the opposite side of this spectrum and doubt it until it's proven beyond a shadow of a doubt. There is, as always, the happy medium.

When getting someone's opinion, beware of the people who have only one side to share, good or bad. The truth usually lies somewhere in the middle; so I keep searching until I find all parts of the perspective pie. Nobody's experience will exactly match your own so try to keep some distance and know your journey will be different. It's essential to educate yourself, but dangerous to hold any one person's opinion as the absolute authority.

To My Beloved
Transplant Coordinator

A letter written two years after my second transplant

Dear Vicky,

There was a time shortly after my diagnosis of chronic rejection that I was completely positive I'd never go through another lung transplant. I'd had my shot at life, I was going to die and that was okay. I think I'd been dealing with the disease for about a year when it hit me I wanted to do anything I could to try and stay on this planet a little longer. I still had things I wanted to do! That's when I decided to make an appointment to talk to the team about getting a second transplant.

I did just that. I met with the head surgeon and he explained the elevated risks of a second go-round. After that I met with your predecessor, Betty. She told me horror stories about second transplants in general and how I shouldn't even bother. She said it was a bad idea and that I should put it out of my mind. I went home and prepared to die without hope of another life-saving surgery.

Months later Betty quit and you came on board. I was home when you called me to introduce yourself but I didn't answer the phone. By that point I didn't really see what more the team could offer me and I avoided contact. I listened to your voice over the answering machine and had very little interest in getting to know this new transplant coordinator.

When I came in for my next appointment at the clinic you were there. I was very angry because I didn't understand why I needed to drag myself, my oxygen tanks and all my tubing over to the hospital when I was dying and there wasn't anything more that could be done. From my position, getting there was difficult, being there was pointless and getting home was exhausting. I resented those visits and was cantankerous towards all who entered my little exam room. You were no exception.

That's what is so mysterious to me, even to this day. How did you do it? How did you walk into the room, encounter my snarling and spitting, and see right past it? How did you look inside me and see my pain, hurt and fear? Could you somehow see how desperately I wanted to live? What made you decide to fight for me and help me get on the list for a second transplant?

I have no answers to these questions. What I know is that you moved a few mountains out of the way and cleared the path for me to pursue my dream of living another day. It's because of you and your instincts to help me that I'm here, two new lungs and years later. It's because of you that I've been able to fall in love with the man of my dreams. It's because of you that I'm able to write my book. It's because of you that I'm able to breathe in spring, fall, winter and summer. It's because of you that I look forward to another tomorrow.

How do I properly express gratitude for the monumental role you have played in my entire existence? There simply is no way.

I'm not alone in this dilemma. How many people can say these same words to you? How does that feel, to have made such a dramatic impact on so many lives?

May all the compassion you've shown to others be given to you when you need it most. My passionate hope is that your own joy will be proportionate to the love you've given to so many patients.

Thank you so much for moving here and taking Betty's place. No more post-it notes!

With all my breath,
Tiffany

Mistakes, Mistakes, Mistakes

We expect a lot from our health care providers. Perfection, in fact. They're never allowed to make mistakes, and if they do, we sue them for all we can get. We hold them to extremely high and sometimes paradoxical standards. For example, I want my surgeon to have a soft bed-side manner but, equally, I want him to exude the kind of confidence that would never make me doubt his competence. More over, I want him to be equipped with an ego that would not allow *him* to ever doubt his own competence. For one individual to possess the proper inner balance that would be required for both gentleness and a very high opinion of oneself … well, that would be a very unique individual indeed.

In short, patients and families often expect the impossible. There's nowhere to go from there except to anger and disappointment. The truth is, mistakes *will* happen in medical settings. Doctors are only humans, right?

There's a fine line between an honest mistake and unacceptable negligence. It's important to define these two for yourself. When a mistake is made, you have a choice on how you'd like to handle it.

Bloody Mess:

During one of my hospital stays, I was dreaming about water. I was all wet and couldn't seem to dry off. Something wasn't right and I eventually pulled myself from the dream into consciousness. Looking down, I could see something shimmering against the dull light from the hallway. I touched my chest and it was cold and sticky. I turned on the bedside lamp to discover my clothes were completely soaked in blood. Panicking, I buzzed my nurse. By the time she arrived, I'd already figured out the problem. My nurse had come in while I was asleep to draw blood out of my Port-a-Cath and failed to properly clamp it off. The line to one of the main arteries in my body had been left open and I was drenched in my own blood.

Amazingly, this didn't seem to have any negative consequences. Perhaps this is why I had no problem forgiving her. After all, it made a great story!

Near But Yet So Far:

I'd been waiting for lungs five years when I got a page at four o'clock on a Tuesday afternoon: they had lungs for me. My family and I rushed to the ER to begin the many-staged process leading up to the operating room. Eventually, we learned that the surgery was "a go" and we celebrated the arrival of my new lungs.

When I woke up after the surgery, nothing was as I had been taught it would be. I was still in the holding area outside of the OR, not ICU. I wasn't intubated. I had an oxygen mask covering my face and I could barely breathe.

When the nurse saw me stirring, she turned on her heels and fetched my surgeon. He sat next to my head and spoke in a quiet, humble tone I'd never heard him use. He explained that I didn't get my lung transplant. While I was under anesthesia, one team was working on me and preparing for the new lungs while the other team was off somewhere else getting the organs to bring home. As the story goes, the cardio-thoracic surgeon took too much of the "tubing" that's essential in properly connecting the heart and lungs. My new lungs simply didn't have much tubing to work with and it made my team nervous.

At this point, I had already been cut open and they were about to take the first lung out. The dilemma: Close me back up and risk that my very sick lungs would never recover from the trauma, or make do with the donor lungs and take on a much more difficult surgery with many complications to overcome. After much discussion, they chose to close me back up and hope that I could survive this set back.

Obviously, I did survive but not without repercussions. Before this incident, I wasn't on oxygen. Afterwards, I was quite disabled and relied on oxygen twenty-four hours a day. This was frustrating and the cause of a few emotional breakdowns.

Despite this unusual and disturbing event, I wasn't angry with my surgeon. Partly, because it didn't seem like his fault. Mostly, because he was so sorry. He didn't apologize once and then give me a pep talk about how it could be worse. He apologized in some way, every time I saw him. Not just for a few weeks, but for a few years. He wasn't being manipulative because he thought I might sue. He was sincerely saddened by what I'd been through. That made all the difference.

Lost But Proud:

A friend of mine had chronic sinusitis. He struggled with it for years and ultimately decided to have sinus surgery. While it's known to be a painful recovery, it's a common procedure and not one he had many worries about. Unfortunately, my friend awoke from this "routine surgery" completely blind in one eye.

The records that were kept by the surgical nurse were upsetting. During the operation, no attending was present. The entire procedure was done by a young resident. Apparently, the resident found himself "lost" inside the sinus cavity, and, instead of stopping and calling in help, he decided to continue poking around. He poked around so long that he eventually broke through the sinus wall and severed the optic nerves. The sinuses were never cleaned out and my friend spent the next few months visiting eye specialists who concluded there was no way to repair the damage.

In speaking to other ENT doctors I've learned that it's not unusual for someone who's inexperienced to get lost inside the sinus. What is inexcusable is that the doctor didn't call in an attending. My friend lost his eye because of one person's unwillingness to ask for help. In this case, the doctors were sued. After a few years, my friend was awarded some money for his suffering. I think, if he had a choice, he would rather have his eye instead of the cash.

What I Know Now:

I used to be a student in cosmetology school. My hands would shake and I'd feel sick at the idea of having someone's *hair* in my hands. What if I gave them a bad hair cut? How could I live with myself?? And, in fact, when I did ruin somebody's hair, I spent many sleepless nights worrying about her and wishing I could go back in time and fix it all.

That said, I can't even begin to fathom the feeling of having someone else's life in your hands. I couldn't do it. As a patient, sometimes I forget to give my caregivers credit for the magnitude of what they do.

While it's true that we should hold our doctors to a high standard, when does that standard become too high and therefore counter-productive? While there certainly must be repercussions for irresponsible or reckless physicians, I can't help but ask myself some questions. If we lived in a society where we were more willing to accept the possibility of human error, would doctors be more likely to admit a mistake? I can't help but wonder how different things might be if they felt safe in speaking up about an error instead of feeling the need to cover up.

As a patient I must let go of unrealistic expectations. Doctors are human. I also must take responsibility for what I can protect myself against. When and if honest mistakes are made, I must practice forgiveness. There's nothing to gain by hating them.

As caregivers, there must be a value placed on honesty and humility. I'm much more likely to understand a mistake if it's approached directly rather than hidden or underplayed.

In many ways, technology has moved faster than our consciousness. We continue to carry the old perceptions of doctors as gods and infallible. Therefore, when they do fall, we're outraged and feel victimized. The truth is, we're living in a new age of medicine where much can be done and much can go wrong. There's a time and a place for lawsuits but there's also room for accepting the risks that come along with our modern miracles.

A Letter to Medical School Administrators

A letter written after I'd given several talks to med students and met similar responses

To Whom It May Concern:

Every time I speak to a group of med students I get the same question: "How are we supposed to be able to care for patients with respect and compassion when the system's continually pushing us for results, not quality of time spent?" It's a good question and one I've come to dislike.

There's no doubt that our medical system isn't set up for doctors to be personal therapists. They're under great pressure to do the job and do it quickly. I also think we have missed the point.

When it comes to patient care, one option is to sit down and engage in a heart-to-heart with great depth and emotion. The other option, often taken, is to ignore a patient's emotional state and try to push past it long enough to get the answers needed in order to treat the physical problem.

There is a middle ground. Fake it. Good patient care doesn't have to be the result of a bleeding heart. Using good assessment skills and a basic understanding of human emotion, doctors can provide quality care without having to cancel all of the afternoon appointments to spend more time with someone in need.

I don't believe the aspect of patient care that revolves around psychological wellness needs to be in depth or sincere. It can be as rehearsed as all the other doctor-speak taught in med school. It requires observation and practice, two skills that all doctors need, no matter what. Here is my formula for a good bedside manner:

Step One: *See the patient*

When I'm upset about something, I don't usually announce it. That doesn't mean it's not obvious! When doctors come and go and pretend as though life is a bunch of honey lollipops, it makes me more upset. I feel like I'm invisible. That's a desperate feeling.

Step Two: *Acknowledge what you see*
If someone were to acknowledge that they recognize my emotional state, it would calm me down immediately. I'd feel recognized and respected as a human being. Sometimes, this might be all I need.

Step Three: *Ask if there's anything that you, as the doctor, can do to help*
Often there won't be but simply asking is a sign of understanding and compassion—even if you're faking it.

Step Four: *Set boundaries*
This would be about the time that many patients would take up the rest of your afternoon spilling their guts. That's because you've reached out to them and they trust you enough to let some things off their chest. Besides, they most likely have an overload of pent up emotions and you have just opened the floodgates. Let them know you care—even if you don't—but that you have an obligation to the other patients waiting.

Step Five: *Mirror*
Paraphrase what you heard them say and let them know you understand how they could feel that way—even if you don't.

Step Six: *Food for thought*
Let them know you'll mull over the things they've said and will get back with them if you think of anything helpful—even if you won't. This is also a good time to give them names of organizations or individuals that specialize in this part of illness work. Giving them therapists or other support resources can allow them to feel they've left with something that might give them some relief from their current emotional state.
Side Note: This sort of resource list is not something that comes equipped on a standard model physician, but it should. Many patients lack the ability or capacity to seek out help on their own. Many have the ability but just don't know where to look. Either way, you are the one in the world of health care. You are surrounded by recourses every day. All you have to do is organize your list and have it ready for the next person who needs it!

Will this take longer than a normal visit? Perhaps, but not much.
Will this take an emotional toll on the doctor? Not if they learn this as part of a routine visit and can remain emotionally objective and calm.

Will this help patients feel as though they were being treated with respect and kindness? Most certainly.

Will this increase patient compliance? No doubt.

Bedside manner training is quite in vogue. Medical schools all around the country are implementing classes to teach doctors how to have more empathy for their patients. I believe this is an unrealistic goal. You can't teach a person how to feel anything. This will vary from personality to personality, and, with any individual, it will vary from day to day. To attempt to reach this goal is to attempt to hit a moving target; it will happen on occasion but will usually be a miss.

When you're teaching scientific minds, wouldn't it be best to teach a kind of compassion that can be consistent and logical? The truth is, a compassion that's genuine and a compassion that's manufactured are indistinguishable. As a patient, I'd welcome either one.

Your med students don't have to graduate with a degree in sympathy. However, I won't give up on the fight for them to treat me like a whole being and not just a car that needs a tune-up.

It's not that hard. Give them the skills, please, I beg you.

~Tiffany

Practice

Journal entry from June, 2007

During one of my presentations on The Patient Perspective, a surgeon asked me how I thought it was that I was able to get to such a place of peace with illness and death. As much as I'd like to pronounce myself exceptionally deep or terribly smart, the honest answer is simple: practice. Since I was old enough to have even a minor grasp on my disease, I knew I wasn't going to live into my eighties. Or seventies. For that matter, living into my 40's would be a gift. Carlos Castenada has a saying about living with "death on your shoulder." I've lived that way for many, many years.

In several ways and circumstances, I've had the opportunity to practice how I will die. If I were to assess myself, I'd have to admit the first few attempts to die well were not well done. I was riddled with fear. I was in a headlock with denial. I was immersed in self-pity. It wasn't until the third and most difficult time that I was able to move through the stages of grief and arrive in the beautiful place of acceptance and peace. It took practice.

Practice. Isn't that the word doctors use to describe their job? They *practice* medicine. They have a *practice*. It dawned on me when I was answering that surgeon's question that, more than any patient, they're the ones with all the practice in illness and death. They see it every day. They deliver the news that it's time to wrap up life and prepare to say goodbye. They watch it unfold before their eyes in many different ways. They're often present at the moment someone dies.

Why, then, do they lack the answers so many patients want to know? When I was diagnosed with chronic rejection I had one main question; "What do I do now? How should I proceed from here?" The answers I got ranged from a confused shrug to "Well, you're not on oxygen yet!"

Of course doctors and nurses can't tell their patients how to live their lives—or how to die their deaths. They can't give specific, concrete answers on how to feel or what to do. But I can't help but think, considering all their experience, why can't they provide some guidance, a compass to guide the direction of the journey's first steps?

If I could go back in time and tell Tiffany Who Has Just Been Diagnosed With Chronic Rejection And Has No Hope Of A Second Lung Transplant where to go from there, I'd tell her a few things based on what I discovered during my training sessions with dying.

First, she should enjoy the health she has now. I imagine that's what the nurse meant by exclaiming "Well, you're not on oxygen yet."

I'd tell her she has some grieving to do, sadness and anger will be visiting. She'll need to grieve the loss of her future and experience the pain of saying goodbye to those she loves so dearly. It will be tempting to push the grief away but, no matter what, it will find a way to grab you—if only in your dreams. When you push, grief pushes back. The sooner you allow it, the sooner you can move through it.

I'd tell her to think about what's meaningful to her and highlight those parts of her life. If her job's important, keep that job until she can no longer physically do it. If her family's important, make room for them and focus on creating quality time with them as much as possible. If there's something else she always wanted to do, now would be the time to do it, while her body is still able to get around.

Finally, I'd tell her, after the grieving is done, there's a possibility for great inner peace and acceptance of what life has offered. I would offer her information on programs, counselors and other people that might be helpful to her on this journey. I'd tell her I'd answer any question she had about the physical process of her illness and death, whenever she was ready or needed to hear it. I'd promise to be honest with her at every turn, if that's what she wanted.

None of these things I've listed are rocket science. None of these things are terribly deep or complicated. None are too specific, risking misleading her into false fears or hopes. All of these things are simple truths that anyone who spends time with the sick would observe over and over.

This is where being a doctor or nurse becomes very tricky. If you, as a health care provider, aren't willing or interested in exploring the emotional sides of illness, you'll be unprepared to guide your patients in a time of need. If you're not willing to face your own mortality, you'll be uncomfortable dealing with those who are. This is a tall order.

No matter who that patient may be, no matter how difficult or independent, the chances are there'll be a time when they look to their caregiver for guidance. After all, aren't they the ones that do this every day? Aren't they the ones who diagnosed this new twist in the patient's life? Aren't they the ones that understand how this has worked for many others in the past? There's a tremendous opportunity for this caregiver to provide a patient with a confident first step into The Sick World.

From where I sit, doctors and nurses are in an enviable position. They get the honor and privilege of being present at some of the most transformative and pivotal moments in a human life. The question is: Will the practice they get in these moments be something they choose to use or something they choose to deny?

God Willing, I'll be Rich, Dead or Very Sick

Journal Entry from August, 2007

Well, the day has come. I have lost my disability status.

When I started my job last September, my understanding was that I had a nine month work trial period before they would consider whether or not I was "too healthy" and take away my disability.

Well, just as I had feared, I misunderstood the rules. My trial period *actually* started in 1998! Ten years! In ten years, I was allowed to work a total of nine months. They tracked every little job, even before my first transplant. So, that time includes pre-transplant and two lung transplants! How does that make sense? Nine months in ten years? Needless to say, I am past my nine months.

The woman told me that if I had read the gobble-de-gook on their website, I would've known all this. Well, I suppose that's true. And I suppose they try to make it as confusing as possible? Besides that, I spoke to a guy at their office when I started back to work. Why didn't *he* tell me about this? Couldn't he just look at my records and give me a heads up that I only had a few months left of my "trial period"?

And guess what? Here's the best part … they want me to pay them back all the money they gave me this year! That's got to be a joke, right? No. It's not. And, if it were a joke, it would be a very un-funny one.

On top of that, my last day at work is next Friday. Money was going to be tight around here while I tried to make a career out of my public speaking but now … tight sounds like a luxury.

So, I have a big dilemma. I can apply to be reinstated and hopefully avoid having to pay back the thousands and thousands of dollars. I can also have the peace of mind knowing that I will be able to eat and drive my car from A to B.

What I won't be able to do is make one red penny. If I do, those benefits are gone immediately.

I stand on the edge of my future. I have no idea if I will be able to make this book and this voice into a successful livelihood. There is no way to know unless I do it.

Do I take the money and settle for nothingness? Do I give up the money and face possible failure and poverty?

What happens if I become a mediocre success? I may not need that monthly check but I will need my Medicare! Unless I become a millionaire and can buy my own insurance, I can not lose that coverage. God willing, when the time comes for them to take my Medicare away, I will either be rich, dead or sick enough to reapply for disability. What options!
It's all very scary.

Know Thyself!
The Power of Strategic Living

This is a fast-paced world we live in. It's not uncommon for the modern individual to push themselves to pack more and more into one day. We design a string of appointments, errands and work-related tasks that are stacked so carefully, if one part of the string falls behind, we're behind on everything and under great stress to catch up. This kind of effort becomes normal and, if there's a lack of stress, it can feel as though we're not doing enough.

Just because a person gets sick doesn't mean this mentality suddenly stops. The body requires a slower pace but the mind may not recognize this. In order to enhance quality of life and reduce stress, this new mind/body dynamic must be approached consciously.

Slow Going Getting Going:

After thirty-something years of grooming myself, dressing, having breakfast and starting my day, I'd become comfortable with my routine and the time it took to do everything. When I was very ill, like a broken record, I couldn't seem to get it through my head that things had changed and I became chronically late for everything. I hate to be late. At some point I had to face facts: the simple things had become quite difficult. It was time to make the mental adjustment to match my physical reality.

When you become ill, the body no longer has the same level of energy it once did. I could feel the energy being drained from me doing ordinary tasks. I called this energy reserve my gas tank and could clearly visualize when it was full (rarely!), when it was being drained (and by how much) and when it was empty (often!). Like the life regeneration you'll find in a common video game, it takes a time of stillness and quiet to refill the gas tank. It became essential for me to integrate these times of regeneration into my daily routine.

Taking a shower was no longer an option because I couldn't stand up in that kind of heat and still be able to breathe. I had to switch to baths, and baths, by nature, simply take longer. After my bath, I needed time to recover from that exertion. Usually I'd spend around fifteen minutes either lying down or sitting on the edge of my bed. I needed this time to catch my breath and refill my energy's gas tank.

To dress myself, I had to split the task into parts. First, I opened the drawers to the dresser and then had to pause for breath. Bending down was an effort so I moved my clothes to the top drawers and avoided the bottom ones altogether. After catching my breath, I'd pull out the pants, underwear and shirt I wanted to put on. I'd take them over to the bed, and again pause to catch my breath. Sitting down, I'd dress myself, trying to be conscious about going slow. My mind would often forget the limits of my body and I'd perform an action at "normal" speed and pay the consequences with a lengthy recovery. It was astounding how difficult it was to remember to go at my body's pace, not my mind's.

After I'd finish dressing, I spent more time regenerating and gearing up to move back into the bathroom. In the bathroom, I faced some of my most difficult challenges. That's where I brushed my teeth and my hair. The raising of my arms for that length of time was very hard and caused me to get severely out of breath. There was a lot of time spent sitting on the toilet lid and catching my breath during those two tasks.

The next step required a long trip from the bathroom (located in my bedroom) to the kitchen. I'd developed a mental map with different resting spots—I called them stations—along the way. Once I reached the kitchen, there was often a need for a long regeneration period at the kitchen table. This could take as long as a half hour.

Once I'd caught my breath and felt strong enough to stand, I made my way to the cabinet, pulled down a mug, filled it with water and put it in the microwave for 1.5 minutes. This time was another opportunity to sit down and rest. When the bell went off, I wasn't always able to get up at that moment and would feel pressure to recover before my water got cold again. Sometimes I didn't make it in time, and I'd have to reheat the water and try again.

Once the water was hot, I put in a tea bag and made the decision of whether or not I had the breath to walk over to the trash can to dispose of the wrapper. Often, I left it on the counter, deciding it wasn't worth the trip.

Next came the even longer trek to the living room, again taking time to pause at different resting stations. It was often a great effort to make it to the couch, and when I did, it felt like a victory. I set my tea down on the coffee table in front of me and took all the time I needed to recover while watching morning television. By the time I'd caught my breath, the tea had cooled down enough so I could drink it. This felt like an affirmation of the routine's strategy.

It's no wonder I was late to things. With all of this extra effort and time needed to refill the gas tank—and oxygen tank, if I had to leave the house—I usually added an hour or two onto my "normal" regimen. It wasn't until I got realistic about how long things took that I started making my appointments as late in the day as possible and planning appropriately so I had a chance at being on time. I worked to organize my environment to be as accommodating as possible, like putting all of my clothes in the top drawer. As a general rule, I estimated how long it would take me to do something and added on an hour. As I became conscious of my limits, I was better able to strategically set out to accomplish the goals for my day with the least amount of stress and hurry.

Fair Trade:

Quality of life. This is a huge issue when you become ill. There's so much that you have to give up. There's so much that you miss out on. I found that sometimes, to feed my soul, it was worth it to occasionally overdo and pay the consequences. To be irresponsible responsibly, one must plan for the build up and the melt down ahead of time.

One summer, when I was living with chronic rejection, my mother arranged through The Fairy Godmother Foundation for me to meet my favorite singer and then enjoy his concert. They also gave me and my companions a limo ride and a stop off for dinner at my favorite restaurant. This was a very special night I'd never forget—and a night I was way too sick to participate in without repercussions. There was no question in my mind that it was worth it, however, so I began the plans to overdo.

The first step was to clear my schedule two days before and three days after. I made sure I had no doctor's appointments and asked for help with meals and other daily necessities during that time. I rested and rested and rested before the concert. That night, my big oxygen tank was loaded into the limo and my friends and I set out for fun.

Dinner was wonderful. Meeting my favorite singer was awkward but sweet. The concert was just what the doctor ordered. I stood the entire two hours and sang as loud as my crappy lungs would allow. I knew every song. I was flooded with happiness and drank up every minute. When the lights went down and the concert was over, I felt like I'd been hit by a truck.

My friends helped me to the limo and as soon as I we got home, I crawled into bed with all of my clothes on. I stayed in bed for the entire next day. I didn't bathe and I only partially removed what I'd been wearing. I was exhausted and fulfilled. I was able to get out of bed the second day but still didn't have the energy to bathe. By the third day, my tank had enough gas to wash up but I still needed naps and more rest.

I paid the consequences I knew were likely to come from that one night out. It was worth every minute of my three-day recovery. I had filled up with joy and had an experience that would always be close to my heart. Through the fatigue, I could still feel the pulse of the music and, there was no doubt, I'd made a fair trade.

Communication:

The more your loved ones know where you're coming from, the easier things will be for everyone involved. I experience moderate to severe nausea at least once a month, usually more. When I first met my husband, he would try to understand what was happening with me, as it was happening. This created some frustration for both of us because the last thing I wanted to do was talk about nausea when I was nauseous. At the same time, he was worried and really needed for me to communicate what was going on and how he could help. At some point, I got smart and began to educate him on my experiences when I *wasn't* experiencing them.

With the nausea, I explained that talking made me feel more nauseous and talking louder than a whisper was really out of the question. I told him things that could be helpful like, cold compresses, sleep or where to find my nausea medicine. Now, when I get sick like that, he can recognize it, and ask me yes or no questions about which thing I need. He's able to understand me and help me. I'm able to do what I need to do to get through my discomfort more comfortably. By preparing a game plan ahead of time, we were able to work as a team. This brings us both great peace of mind.

Remembering to Remember:

When I was healthy again and had my new set of lungs, I completely abandoned strategic living. Consequently, I found myself in undesirable situations. I was going to work all worn out. I was trying to write at times when I was at my least inspired. I was lacking balance and therefore neglecting parts of my life—like my family—in pursuit of some lofty goal that, in the end, wasn't really important. I had to start taking the lessons of my severe illness and applying them to my healthier life.

One night I was at a party with a bunch of old friends. I was visiting and had to leave the next morning for a long drive home. At home, I had a lot of errands and chores that needed to be done before that Monday, when I was scheduled to work an eleven hour shift.

The party, as many parties do, started getting more interesting as the night wore on. I was getting to know new people, fascinating discussions were cropping up, and those with a few too many drinks were becoming quite entertaining. I really wanted to stay and see how things played out, but I'd promised myself I would leave at midnight. When midnight arrived, I began to negotiate with myself about staying another hour or two. Immediately, I envisioned myself at work on Monday dragging and sick with fatigue. Even as healthy as I was, my gas tank still had its limits. I knew it was time to say goodbye and take care of myself.

Pulling myself away from the party was difficult. My friends teased me about leaving so early and tried to get me to stay. I stood strong, despite my inward protests, and left five minutes after midnight. On the way back to my hotel, the fun of the party faded and I could feel how tired I was. I looked forward to sleep and felt a sense of pride that I was able to override my immediate desires in favor of my future well-being.

The next morning, I awoke refreshed and went for the farewell breakfast. Some of my friends were still sleeping, most of them were hung-over, all of them were tired. I wasn't standing in judgment of their choice to stay at the party, but was relieved to not be in the same situation. I found the stories of the party equally as fun as being there. As difficult as it was to extract myself the night before, I was glad I didn't stay.

I drove home with a clear head, and went to work on Monday with plenty of energy in the tank. I think of this trip often and try to hold onto the lessons I learned when I was so sick, the lessons about being conscious of one's own limits and health strategies. I've learned that self care feels really good and is a strong component to self-love.

What I Know Now:

The realities of illness can be difficult to accept and incorporate into one's life. The fact is, however, the sooner you're able to adjust your daily expectations, the sooner you'll be able to develop strategies that will help you move more efficiently throughout the day. To do this, you must know yourself, your limits and your needs.

Nobody will create a system for you that will maximize your energy and schedule; this is up to you. Nothing is more frustrating than trying to accomplish what you did when you were healthy in the same way now that you're sick. Likewise, the lessons of conscious living and strategizing can be very satisfying when you're of sound body.

The bottom line is to know yourself and love yourself enough to think ahead so you might live life with as much energy in that tank as possible, and with the highest capacity for joy.

Creamy Nougat Filling

Dear Men and Women I've Met Lately,

When I walk down the street carrying an oxygen tank, you stare. When you see the tubes coming from my nose, you stare. You see how skinny I am—size 00—so you stare.

I don't blame you. I really understand. I'd stare too. It must seem so strange, such a mystery. Why would such a young woman be so sick?

When you came up to me in Macy's and told me you'd pray for me, I know you meant for those words to relay your compassion. I couldn't help but wonder, though, how do you know that it isn't *I* that should be praying for *you*?

When you snarled at me in Target and told me I shouldn't have smoked so much, I know you were reacting out of fear. I couldn't help but wonder, though, what are you doing to your body that scares you so much that you see yourself when you look at me?

When you covered your mouth and pointed at me from across the food court, I know you didn't think I saw. I couldn't help but wonder, though, how can people be so disconnected from another human being?

This body doesn't represent who I am. My mind and my soul are not sick. My mind and my soul are not tired. They're strong and vibrant and very much alive. This sick body is merely a wrapper that contains a healthy filling.

There was a time when my tank and my tubes embarrassed me. There was a time when your stares made me want to run and hide. Now I know that if you take a moment to see past the accoutrements and look in my eyes, you'll see who I am. The decision is yours. I can't control whether you choose to see me or see my tubes. All I can do is know who I am and let it shine through.

Equally, when I look at you, I have the same choice to make. I hope I choose to see past your wrapper and look in your eyes.

Looking forward to seeing you soon,
The Skinny Girl with the Oxygen Tank Who has a Creamy Nougat Filling

Goodbye Training Wheels

Journal entry from September, 2007

So far, the vast majority people I have told about my disability status being "revoked" have simply freaked out. Panic on their faces. Fear in their voice.

Is there something I don't know?
Why am I the only one who seems to think I might be able to live without it?
Their fear makes me doubt my tentative confidence.

I have said for so long that I aspired to stand on my own two feet.
I had a goal of becoming financially independent down the road. It looks like Social Security has decided to make that a reality a little sooner than I had planned it out to be.

Nonetheless, I want to take the training wheels off at some point … why not now?

Look out world! If you see me coming on my ten speed, please move out of the way because I just took the training wheels off and I'm not sure how to steer this thing!

The Emotional Maze

There's little in this world that can turn your life upside down like illness can. Whether you are home with the flu or facing serious disease, emotional adjustments will need to be made in order to accommodate the unwelcome guest.

This part of the medical revolution involves being proactive in your own emotional journey so that you'll eventually find your way to a richer, deeper understanding of your true inner self.

Winding your way through the emotional maze can be disorienting and challenging. What you'll find at the end, though, is that it's possible to love life no matter how difficult it becomes.

The Sick World and The Well World

There was a time when I was honored to be a member of a very private world. I call this The Sick World. This is a place that's filled with people who are living their lives day to day, doctor appointment to doctor appointment, and grappling with all that it means to be alive. When you live in The Sick World, there's a certain understanding among its residents. There's a depth to this community, a vibrating knowledge of the fragility and value of life. I'm proud to say that I once lived in The Sick World. This same understanding is difficult to find when you're out in The Well World.

When I lived in The Sick World, I was no longer interested in what I once was. It was as if I had moved to another planet. I didn't care about who was playing in the Super Bowl or which celebrity was dating another celebrity. I didn't even care much about the state of the country, since it rarely had an impact on my little universe. People would tell me their problems and I could see with an indescribable understanding just how and why they were standing in their own way. It was as if I'd been given a map to living; it all seemed so obvious. The only problem was that I didn't have the physical ability to engage in it very much myself.

That level of insight could be satisfying and my level of non-attachment to the dramas of this life were freeing. However, it was also stressful for me when visitors from The Well World approached, expecting me to care about all the things they cared about and to the same degree. Few people spoke, or even understood, my language, the language spoken in The Sick World. I've created two lists to help illustrate how different the focus is in each world.

The Top 10 Things Occupying the Thoughts of People in the Well World:

1. Family/Children
2. Marriage—getting it, keeping it, dissolving it
3. Job/Money
4. Physical Appearance
5. Traveling
6. Body—exercise, diet
7. Friends—socializing and gossiping
8. Entertainment—where should we go tonight?
9. State of the world, politics
10. Hobbies

My Top 10 List of Thoughts Occupying my Mind when I lived in the Sick World:

The top 4 are the same, but with a slight twist.

1. Family/Friends and how they will cope with my death
2. Marriage—surviving w/less conflict, dealing with feeling trapped
3. Body—worry, constant inventory, acute awareness
4. My physical appearance—embarrassment over carrying my oxygen tank and tubes
5. tairs—things like stairs and inclines began to become a part of how I planned my day. If I knew there were stairs where I was going I'd to give myself plenty of extra time to get up them, or find an alternate route.
6. Appointments—the landmarks of my life!
7. Getting to another room, getting food
8. A conversation
9. TV
10. My feelings

When I look at those lists now, I can feel sad for myself that I lived in The Sick World. It seems so small from The Well World vantage point. There's a certain depth and truth to The Sick World, but I don't suggest people who are living in The Sick World have chosen that address, nor would they be happy to be a permanent resident. Those that live in The Sick World usually strive to return to The Well World. I envied those who occupied time contemplating buying a new house or where they would go on the next vacation. There were times I resented the simplicity of my life and yearned for the complexity of The Well World.

Despite its hardships, there's something to be said for a world where That Which Is Important remains clear and is always at the surface. It's my challenge now to somehow hold on to some of the clarity of the Sick World while enjoying the physical freedom of The Well World. This is a challenge I've often failed to meet. There's beauty and heartache in both worlds. The trick is learning from each other and valuing what we have right now.

To all of those living in the private, misunderstood Sick World, may your whispers be heard so that others can learn about That Which is Important. To all of those living in the dominant and often oblivious Well World, may you open your eyes to the lessons of The Sick World and slow down, calm down and always appreciate the deep breaths you're able to take.

The Diagnosis

There are pivotal moments in everyone's life when something happens and they are no longer headed in the same direction they were only moments before. This can happen when you fall in love, when you get a new job, or when you're diagnosed with a new illness.

Changing Parental Hopes:

I was too young to remember my first diagnosis of cystic fibrosis. I was six months old and wasn't going to the bathroom properly. This tipped off the doctors and they did a sweat test on me that came back positive for CF.

I'll never forget the story my mother told me of her reaction. In fact, its image is so burned into my brain that I feel like I have a memory of it. She said that when she got home from the doctor she held me and cried for hours. She just wandered around the house whispering over and over, "My baby, my baby." I was the fourth child, and my mother felt sure she'd worked out most of the child-rearing kinks and I was to be "the perfect child." My diagnosis took this dream away and changed both of our lives forever.

There's such a void of knowing when you're in the early stages of facing an illness like CF. Learning all the new medications, all the ways to administer them and figuring out what possibilities the future may hold is overwhelming, to put it mildly.

At the time of my diagnosis, the life expectancy of a CFer was around twelve years old. My mother decided she'd compensate for my short and difficult life by never refusing me anything. This approach worked fine until she noticed I'd become a raging brat by the age of six! She started reining me in at that point and saved me from myself.

While I was too young to remember my diagnosis, in its own way, it was a third parent to me. As I grew up my understanding of mortality and illness evolved along with me. I can not remember a time when I did not ponder these things—even at an age when I could barely grasp the concepts. Through time, the diagnosis and the illness have been my greatest teacher.

As for my parents, I feel a tremendous sadness when I think of that time in our lives—how scary it must have been for them and how many parental hopes for my life they must have had to throw away. As much as my life has been a roller-coaster, they've ridden it with me the entire way. Being the parent of a sick child never ends.

Sugar Momma:

It had been about six months since I had received my first set of donor lungs. I started being consumed with thirst; my thoughts were often occupied with visions of tasty beverages. Second to cold drinks, my desires centered around long naps. If I wasn't day dreaming about lemonade, I was pondering the softness of my sheets and counting the minutes until I could curl up and sleep.

Along with my day dreams, nausea and stomach pains went on for weeks until I went in for a clinic visit. It was then I was diagnosed with diabetes. I knew this was a possibility because of the steroids I was taking, but I was floored nonetheless. I was overwhelmed with all of the new information and injection regimens.

During the time of this diagnosis, I had also been preparing to go back to college. There was already an element of feeling overloaded but this new development pushed me over the edge. To be honest, I freaked out. I called the school and told them, through uncontrollable sobs, that I would not be returning after all. Transplant had been plenty to handle. Adding in diabetes just seemed like a nightmare.

In time, diabetes became just another part of my life. When I look back on my conversation with the college administrator I feel pretty embarrassed. From where I sit now, it certainly wasn't worth that level of drama! At the time, that diagnosis appeared like a mountain too high to climb. Now, it just looks like a bump in the road.

From Panic to Peace:

When I received my diagnosis of chronic rejection, it was two years post-transplant and I was twenty-nine years old. My lung function had been falling and, after countless tests, the transplant team ruled out every other possibility. They made a clinical diagnosis of the illness and, despite my dropping numbers, I was completely shocked. I really didn't know much about chronic rejection except that it killed you. And that's less the case now, there are more things that can be done to treat it.

My initial reaction was one of cold panic. I felt a wave of nausea pass through me and I fought to stay focused on what the doctors were saying. I felt like I was underwater and I could barely make out their words. I don't think I cried about it right away, even after I got home. All I could feel was fear and confusion; sadness hadn't made its way to the top yet.

The only thing I wanted to know was "What do I do now?" Should I quit working even though I don't feel that poorly yet? Should I pretend like nothing happened and just forge onward as usual? How long do I have? How will I die? What will it feel like when things get worse? How do I live with this new information? Could this really be happening so soon after my transplant?

The new diagnosis knocked the wind out of me and it took a long time before I could stand up again. No matter how long I've lived with illness, there seems to be a never ending supply of surprises.

What I Know Now:

One minute we're sick, getting tests and hoping it's something that's easily treatable so that we don't have to take too much time out of our lives to deal with it. The next minute that sickness has been made into a diagnosis, our busy lives drop away, and all we want to do is survive. Making that mental and emotional transition is arduous and tangled. I can't really think of anything else in this world that's changed my life as dramatically as a new diagnosis. There's a great loss that comes from letting go of the things that illness takes away. The hope I can offer is that there's an opportunity, after the mourning, to learn profound lessons of life and self.

Brave

My grandmother calls me "the brave one." That word seems to be applied to me a lot these days. At first I found it to be a nice compliment. Now, it makes me angry.

I'm not brave. I cry and fall apart, I just don't often do it in front of you. What would it look like to you if I were not brave? Would I sit in the corner of the room rocking back and forth? Would I stop speaking? Would I just die?

I don't know how to be anything other than what I am. I put one foot in front of the other, every day. Sometimes my steps are steady, other times I fall into a pothole of darkness. I get scared. I get sad. I worry. I'm not brave. I'm just getting through it.

Sometimes I think they call me brave because it takes the pressure off of them. If I'm brave then I'm okay, taking care of myself, not needing support. If I'm brave, they don't need to find a way to give me strength. If I'm brave they can walk away without guilt.

Finding the Dragon Shrinker

One of the greatest challenges of being ill is finding someone to talk to about what you're truly experiencing. When I was very sick, I was surrounded by people who loved me, but I was overwhelmed by the belief that I couldn't be completely honest with them about my deepest thoughts and emotions. My feelings were complicated and heavy, too heavy to be confessed to those I loved. I simply didn't want them to carry my burdens.

This is why I sought out a good therapist. I needed to talk to someone who could handle my situation, and who better than a professional? What I eventually found was that a good therapist can save your life and a bad one can make it worse.

The Silent Treatment:

I was only sixteen but I wanted to talk to someone about having CF. I needed to process my thoughts about dying and my feelings of being different. My parents got me a shrink and I began to see him once a week.

Despite my deep desire to talk, I was an ornery teenager and was unwilling to open myself up to just anyone. This therapist had the Stare-at-the-Patient-Until-They-Talk approach and I had the Stare-at-the-Therapist-Until-He-Impresses-Me approach. We weren't a good team. We spent many sessions with only a greeting and farewell passing between us.

At some point, he made the bold move of asking me a question. He wanted to know how I felt about having this disease. I believe my answer was along the lines of "It's fine." He went on to praise me for how well I handled it—based on that answer—and told me I was a model patient. I thought he was a complete idiot but, at the time, I always accepted any compliments I could get so I didn't bother to correct him. I stopped going to see him shortly after that session.

Who Is the Patient Here?:

I was in my early twenties and getting ready to go off to an acting conservatory. My illness was progressing, I was worried about my mortality and, once again, I felt the need to process my feelings with someone outside my inner circle. My doctor recommended a therapist who specialized in treating people with illness. This thrilled me and I began to see her on a regular basis. At first I liked her. She made me cry about stuff which I took as a good sign. After seeing her for over a year, however, I started noticing that some of her advice was way off the mark. I became wary of what she told me and lost some trust in her perspective.

During one of our sessions I was talking about my life, I think I was crying again, and she began to interrupt me to tell me stories from her life. It was very jarring but I tried to see how they related. Simply put, they didn't relate. She was a person who had suffered sexual abuse as a child and one day she decided she wanted me to know it. It was almost as if she had gotten sick of listening to me and decided she wanted me to listen to her for a change.

She talked for the remainder of the hour and I left feeling like I never had the right to complain about anything ever again. Clearly, she was pointing out that my life hadn't been as bad as hers. I felt very uncomfortable when I thought about going back again. I didn't know how to handle it so I canceled my next appointment with a promise to reschedule. I never called her again.

While I feel sad for her, that session made me understand the importance of keeping a professional distance. I needed the illusion that she was healthy enough—strong enough—to handle my emotion. After I saw the man, or woman, behind the curtain I no longer felt comfortable laying my burdens at her feet. It is for this reason that I try to remain on a professional level with my therapists and resist the urge to learn much about their personal lives.

Help Arrives:

When I was diagnosed with chronic rejection after my first transplant, I was confused, scared and devastated. I couldn't believe I'd been given this tremendous gift and the ride was over already. Perhaps more than any other time in my life, I needed to talk to someone.

A friend of a friend recommended Tom to me and I hoped he could help me work through some of my pain. Tom did much more than that. He became my rock, my teacher and my sanity. I have countless stories I could tell about a time when Tom took me from a very dark place and helped me transform my perspective and my life. I couldn't begin to describe how valuable he's been to me over the years. Because one story is no less valuable than the next, I'll simply tell you the story of our first meeting that I still think about to this day.

It was difficult to even tell my story to this stranger without tears. I was going through so much and needed guidance so desperately. I told Tom of my fears and my fear of my fears. He listened and commented as I spoke. When I'd come to a resting point, he pulled a book off of his shelf. I don't remember what it was called but it was a paperback children's book with an orange dragon on the cover. Tom presented the book to me as if I were in a group of kindergarten children. He sat the book on his lap so that I could clearly see the pages from my seat while he slowly read and turned the pages. At first this made me feel silly and uncomfortable but, like a kindergartener, I quickly became immersed in the book and forgot myself.

Tom told me the story of a young boy who found a little orange dragon and wanted to keep him as a pet. The little boy would show his pet to his mom and she would respond with "There are no such thing as dragons." For some reason, the dragon grew bigger and bigger. The boy showed the pet to his father and was again given the response, "There are no such thing as dragons." Still, the dragon grew bigger. One day the father came home from work to find that the house was bursting open. The dragon had grown so large his head was poking through the roof and his limbs were hanging out of the windows. The father was very upset and asked the boy where this dragon came from. The boy told him it had been in the house all along. The dragon then began to shrink and soon was, once again, the size of a small dog.

As the dragon, the boy, the mother and the father cuddled on the sofa, the mother wondered why the dragon had gotten so large. The boy answered, "I don't know. I suppose he just wanted to be acknowledged."

I quickly found the value of this story as Tom and I began tackling my own dragons. I was astounded at how quickly they shrunk when I had the strength to look at them and truly acknowledge their existence. This concept laid the groundwork for all of our sessions. To this day, Tom and I face my dragons head on and, after the initial fear of their power, marvel at how quickly they become small.

I believe so strongly in the importance of Tom's role in my life that I'm unsure if I would still be here today without his guidance through the dragons of terminal illness and recovery.

What I Know Now:

Finding a good therapist isn't easy. Just because someone has a degree doesn't make them worthy of being a key player in the complexities of your life. Shop for the right one and don't be afraid to move on if something doesn't feel right. I wish everyone luck in finding the right professional to help you shrink your dragons, whatever they may be.

Around Any Corner

Journal entry from December, 2004

Hope is attachment in disguise.
Around any corner there may lurk a monster.
Around any corner there may lurk an angel of mercy.

To hope for the angel only makes finding a monster all the more terrifying.
To be resigned to finding a monster saps any possibility of experiencing joy as you make your way to the next corner.

Do not hope.
Do not decide all is lost.

Rather than wait until you turn the corner to discover the monster or the angel, seek them out now.
Make them come to you, on your terms.

Befriend the monster—inspect his warts and make peace with the fear he provokes within you.
While it is certain his face will still startle you from time to time, if he becomes a familiar companion you will grow immune to his roar.

The angel of mercy may at first appear to be an embodiment of the ideal.
Her beauty may mesmerize you but, upon deeper inspection, she too is flawed.
Befriend her also and speak to her of what you desire.

You will find mercy and monsters come in many forms.
In fact, if you look hard enough, you might discover that monsters and angels have no differences at all.
They are one in the same.

Transplant Should Be Illegal

Journal entry from June, 2002

Elizabeth Kubler-Ross's stages of grief are well known in our modern society. We all know that denial, anger, sadness, bargaining and acceptance cycle through us as we're processing loss. What do those stages look like though? Would we really know them when we see them in another's behavior? Better yet, would we be able to recognize them when we, ourselves, are in the middle of one of these emotional cycles? Recently, I've found that, while the description is simple and obvious, the manifestation can be deceptive.

It was about a month ago that I was sitting in my therapist's office, telling him about my new realization. I'd come to the conclusion that transplant, while having its good points, was primarily destructive and cruel. Because of this, my passionate belief was that transplant should be made illegal. After all, it was unnatural and only provided the patients with a limited extension of their lives. I plotted my moves to take on the fall of organ transplantation.

It sounds so silly to me now. No, it sounds sad. Looking back, it's so obvious I was in a stage of anger and looking for a scapegoat to absorb my emotion. What's startling is that I had no idea that was what was happening. I truly believed I'd found my new political calling: a large scale wrong had been done and I needed to find a way to expose the flaws in the system. I spoke passionately and logically. I had plenty of reasons to support my position. I had no idea I was externalizing a very internal grief.

I turned on the news today and I heard a mother making a passionate plea. Her daughter had fallen overboard from a cruise ship and died. She was declaring that, while we think that cruises are safe, they really aren't. She was calling for stricter laws and protocols around all cruise ships. People were listening to her. Arguments were being made for and against the safety of cruise ships. What I saw was her stage of grief. She was angry about her loss and looking for the scapegoat, just like I was. It was fascinating that people were listening to her arguments and not seeing past them to her pain.

Cruises are actually relatively safe. Transplant shouldn't be illegal. Care must be taken when listening to the diatribes of the grieving. What may seem like a logical argument may just be the manifestation of a grief searching for something to blame.

When we're anticipating the stages of grief in those who've suffered loss, do we really know what we're looking for? When we're in the middle of our own grief pain, do we really know what's driving us? Despite all of our psychological sophistications, I believe that answer is very often no.

The Lazy Scale

I know a girl who was waiting for a transplant and, like most of us, she was very ill. She and her mother were tightly wound together and her mother went with her everywhere. I remember a day when the girl was in the waiting room with a soda sitting on a table directly in front of her. She turned to her mother and asked her to hand her the drink can. I was astounded that her mother obliged and reached over her daughter to lean forward and hand her the soda that was nearly within arm's reach.

I also know a girl who had just had chemo, had contracted a terrible lung infection and insisted on going to work anyway. She didn't want to be a "wimp."

There are two sides to the Lazy Scale and it's not always easy to know which way to tip it.

Lazy Slob:

I don't know that you could ever call me wimpy but you certainly could get away with calling me spoiled. Growing up, I had very few domestic chores due to my illness. My mother waited on me in hopes that, making things like eating convenient, I'd do more of it. When I was sick, my parents would move heaven and earth to get me what I wanted just to make me feel better, even for a second. I've also observed this same dynamic in many of my chronically ill friends.

Today, I do very little around the house. My husband does the vast majority of cleaning, laundry and cooking. There are times when I'll pass on doing something because it requires me to get off the couch. I've battled a shopping addiction that put me in about $10,000 of debt because I didn't know how to tell myself "no" when I really wanted that new shirt or pair of shoes.

I'm aware that none of this is making me look very good. I can only hope that my confessions here haven't made you so disgusted that you close the book and walk away. The reality is that these patterns were established so early in life that I've had to work very hard to break them.

There's a fine line between indulging oneself because you're sick and crossing that line into entitlement. There have been areas where I've been able to change my ways: I no longer shop as though I'm rich. I worked hard to take away my underlying belief that I deserve whatever material thing I see because it's shiny, I want it and I've had a hard life. I'm no longer in debt and it's been that way for many years. As for helping around the house … well, let's just say I'm a work in progress.

In my daily life, I'm very driven and unbelievably lazy at the same time. I often beat myself up for the lazy part, but, at other times, I think I'm being too harsh and excuse it as "relaxing." Because of my history, I can often have internal arguments about which way I fall on the Lazy Scale. Neither side is usually the victor; confusion wins.

Working Slob:

There's a flip side on the Lazy Scale. There's the part of me—and I've also observed this pattern in many of my chronically ill friends—that will take on too much and meet demands that need not be met.

This is especially evident when it comes to my job. There have been times when I was in full-blown pneumonia and still insisted on going to work. There have been times when I was experiencing acute rejection and I scheduled my injections of massive doses of IV steroids around my work schedule. Keep in mind, these were not jobs in which I was responsible for saving the world. These were low-paying receptionist jobs, deli clerk jobs or pet sitting jobs. For all of these, it would have been perfectly acceptable to call in sick—but, somewhere inside of me, I believe that the delicate balance of the universe will crumble if I stay home from work one day.

There's a feeling inside of me that, in order to play the role of working person, I must never succumb to illness. Perhaps this comes from a feeling of inadequacy. Perhaps this comes from a fierce loyalty to my employer. Perhaps this comes from a deep resistance to admitting my physical short-comings. My guess is that it's a combination of all of these.

What I Know Now:

There's a strange dichotomy that pulls at those of us who have lived a long time with illness. There are the patterns that keep us from becoming fully independent and those that encourage us to push beyond a necessary limit. All that we can do is work to unravel the patterns that keep us from fully engaging in our lives and focus on how to care for ourselves when the body needs rest and healing.

Beautiful Witness

Journal entry from September, 2006

When I was dying, I didn't have the physical ability to take care of my dog. I wouldn't have been able to walk him, play with him or feed him at consistent times. Because of this, he lived with my parents. I missed him specifically, and, in a more general sense, I missed having an animal presence in the house. My solution to this was to get a bird.

I'd never had a bird before and didn't know much about them. I did a fair amount of research and settled on getting a cockatiel. I was hoping to get a boy because the boys sing and talk while the girls squawk one repetitive note. When they're babies, there's no way to tell if they're male or female without a blood test, which I wouldn't do to a poor baby bird. Instead, I chose a rather unfortunate technique for determining the gender. I took out all of the birds in the store and looked for the meanest one; I figured that would be the boy. There was one that certainly fit the bill. This bird didn't back down or fly away. When I went to pick him/her up the bird bit at me and hissed. It may seem bizarre, but this is the bird that I took home!

She wasn't a he. She was a female and the meanest one at that! For this reason, I named her Spike. She didn't like me but she did like my boyfriend at the time, whom she allowed to pet her and hold her. Me, she would rather just bite and fly away. It would be an understatement to say we weren't best friends.

Despite this, however, that bird was a key piece of my life. She was my constant companion in the quiet, lonely world of my living room. I'd watch her with wonder and interest as she went about her day. She was allowed to fly around and I loved watching her at the window perch, communing with the trees and outside birds. Sometimes, her squawking would make me crazy. Often, it made me laugh. She was easy to care for and a joy to live with.

Today, I don't watch my bird very much. I'm busy with my life and my two dogs. She interrupts my phone conversations with shrieks of joy and I find that annoying. She still communes with the trees and outside birds and I find that

110

amusing. She doesn't get out of her cage much because my whippet would like to eat her for lunch. Amazingly, she really doesn't seem to mind. She still hisses at me but loves my husband. Her role in my life is no longer center stage, but more one on the sidelines.

Sometimes I feel guilty that Spike has taken a back seat in my life. She gave me so much at the time I needed it most. Occasionally, I wonder how a bird this ornery could have meant so much to me at any time, no matter the circumstance.

There's a deep and meaningful gift that animals give us. When I was dying, Spike certainly made this contribution ten-fold. That gift was being my witness. She was a conscious, living being that saw me at the times when I was at my most raw, my most real and my most vulnerable. I was alone, but with my bird. I never held back my tears to prevent Spike from being uncomfortable. I never hesitated to display how sick I felt to allay her worry. I never wondered if she could handle the depth of my situation. Spike remained squawking and busy throughout all of my ups and downs. She was my beautiful witness and, for this reason, her little spirit will always be bound to mine … whether she bites me or not.

Worry

Journal entry from August, 2000

I woke up this morning with my lower back hurting and an aching down my legs. It's been going on a few days now. Of course, I'm worried. What if I'm starting to go into kidney failure?

Later in the day, I noticed I was spontaneously sighing a lot. What does that mean? Is that a sign of rejection? Am I losing lung function?

Also, I'm tired of being tired. Am I ever going to feel energetic? Will my life always be like walking through a swamp just to get from A to B? Is my fatigue normal? Is it all in my head? Is it something I could overcome if I pushed myself harder? Is there something wrong with me?

I'm weary of the internal evaluation I'm constantly doing regarding my body. I want to be free to think of other things. I want to live a life in which each tingle, twinge and pang isn't a cause for concern and anxiety. What must it be like to have a body that functions without all of these warning bells?

Why Am I Crying—Really?

There's a point at which emotions and body chemistry intertwine and that can make life very confusing. There was a time when I was on high alert to my emotions. If I cried or felt depressed, I diligently sought out a reason with intent to "fix" it. Over time, I've learned that there may not be a reason and there may be no need for fixing anything. Instead of reacting to my intense emotions, I more often ask myself, "Why am I feeling this way, really?"

Hormonally Challenged:

When I was in my mid-twenties, there was a period of about one week in which I cried—no sobbed—most of the day, every day. That doesn't sound like a long time, but it felt like months. I was completely disabled by my emotions. I'd fluctuate from a few tears to hysterics. I had friends whom I'd call and cry to on a regular basis. Some of them tried their best to assign a good reason to my distress. The theories were astounding!

A popular theory, and one I attempted to work with, was that I was grieving the future loss of my lungs. I was preparing to move back home for my transplant, and, therefore, I was unconsciously sad about the prospect of my body parts being replaced. Yes, we were grasping at straws. The emotion was out of control, however, and there was desperation to hone in on the problem and resolve it.

One night, I was sobbing in my bed. I thought I was losing my mind. I got up and began to get dressed. It was time to check myself into the funny farm. I needed help and I couldn't stand the mysterious angst any longer. Ultimately, however, I chose to put off the funny farm, got back in bed and decided I'd start by calling a therapist in the morning.

I got a few names from my CF doctor and placed a few frantic calls to local psychologists. None of them called me back. What's up with that? I was left to my own devices.

I don't know what made me think of it. I don't know how the bell went off in my head. Nonetheless, like a light bulb in a dark room, it dawned on me that all of these problems had started around the time I began taking birth control. I called my gynecologist and spoke with her. She explained I must have a problem with estrogen withdrawal. I'm fine when I'm on the pill, but when I take the sugar pill, during the week of my cycle, my body reacts to the lack of estrogen. In short, my hormones were making me crazy. I can't tell you how much I wished I'd been informed of *that* possible side effect ahead of time!

I could've tried to assign reasons to that intense emotion for the rest of my life. Truth is, there was no exterior provocation, and, therefore, no true reason would ever be found.

Sleeping Beauty:

As much as I want to interact and enjoy myself, I just can't physically find the energy. As much as I'd like to be able to engage in conversation, my brain is simply out of order and I can't form clear thoughts. As much as I'd like to smile, my mouth is too heavy and it remains flat.

This is how depression feels. This is how fatigue feels. This has been a part of my illness.

For so much of my life, I've thought of myself as a somber person. I've labeled myself serious, dull and dark. That is, before I started getting more sleep. The difference in my personality when I'm sleep-deprived and when I'm not is striking. My body needs more sleep than the eight to nine hours a night suggested by the experts. If I miss some sleep, I must make up for it with naps. If I don't, I will quickly fall back into my fatigue and depression.

There were so many years that I was unaware of this need. Instead, I went about labeling and identifying myself by the behaviors that manifest when I was just exhausted. Today, with consistent and sufficient rest, my husband thinks of me as "one of the happiest people he's ever known." I still laugh when he says that. It's so hard to see myself in a different, cheerful light.

Crabby-Puss:

After a bronchoscopy, I usually spend the rest of the day sleeping off the drugs they gave to sedate me through the procedure. Beware to those who pass by the bed of Crabby-Puss!

Those medications make me so ultra-sensitive that even the slightest noise is like nails on a chalkboard. I have been known to yell at my mother for "walking too hard" or "eating those loud crackers."

It's imperative to keep a list of the medications that make me crazy and how. I know now that Prednisone makes me angry, certain anti-nausea meds make me hallucinate and allergy meds will make me pass-out with no warning. Tracking these things is important for me and even more important for those who dare to be near me!

What I Know Now:

There are so many things that can affect our mood: Sleep. What we ate. Medications. Hormonal cycle. Blood sugar. Pain. And yet, it's often our inclination to search for an emotional source instead of considering a physiological one. While I'm a huge advocate for dealing with emotions, there are some feelings that will only pass with time or a physical adjustment. Did you know that it's possible to cry as a release without assigning a meaning to the tears? I didn't.

To act on physiological emotions can prove hazardous to one's life. How many times have I decided that my feelings were related to a person, had a fight with them, and then regretted my words once my physical state resolved? Too many!

It's important to pay attention and consider biochemical reasons for emotions, especially when you're dealing with illness. Unfortunately, you can't make negative feelings disappear with your desire. You can, however, allow them without needing to act on them. Often, discovering that an intense feeling is coming from your physical state, and not a problem with your life, can be a relief. That alone can help to calm the storm. Regardless, one must hunker down and wait for the storm to pass without doing too much damage to your life in the meantime!

Fear

(roughly one week after surgery)

Journal entry from April, 2004

Well, the day that we were never sure would come did arrive. I went through a second transplant a few days ago! I have so much I'm thinking and feeling about that, but I'll have to wait for another time to write it all down.

Today, I want to get down on paper the experience I had immediately before the surgery … before I forget! Amazingly, I've been through the pre-transplant process four times—two transplants and two no-go's—so none of the procedures were much of a surprise. What was different this time, however, was the fear. I was much sicker than before the last transplant, and traveling into mostly uncharted waters by doing this major surgery a second time. My mother was sobbing. She was nearly convinced I wouldn't make it through. From the time I set foot in the ER, I was fighting the pit in my stomach. I tried to be positive but I couldn't deny the fact that this might be the end of me.

When I'd gone through all of the many steps it takes to make it to the holding area—the last step before OR—my fear continued to steadily increase. When we found out the donor lungs were good, I said my goodbyes to my family and was wheeled back to the hallway in front of the OR. The person wheeling me left me alone on my gurney while they went to fetch something. This was the first time since I'd gotten the call that there may be a donor when I'd been completely alone. In this private moment, my fear went through the roof. I was on the verge of panic.

I began talking to myself and trying to soothe my emotions with investigation. Why was I so nervous? What was the root of this terror? It occurred to me I was unconsciously reading a secret cosmic message into my fear. There was a part of me that believed, because I was in fear, that I was making the wrong decision. I was translating my fear into a warning to not proceed with this operation.

As quickly as I realized this, I heard a calming voice in my mind. The voice said, "Just because you fear it doesn't make it wrong." As the sentence repeated, I was able to let go of the part of my anxiety that was related to the belief that fear = run.

When the attendant returned to take me into the operating room, I wasn't without fear. Certainly, I was no longer on the verge of panic, but I still felt sick with worry. All I could do at that point was allow my fear, observe it and remind myself that it wasn't a fortune telling device. I went under anesthesia with fear pulsing through me, and a deep understanding that my fate was up to someone much greater than I or my emotions. It was the truest moment of "Give it to God" I've ever known.

Impermanence Can Be So Deceiving

Journal entry from April, 2007

I've been cranky this week. I haven't been happy with most of the writings I've done for the book. I've been tired. I've declared to my husband a few times that I was depressed.

I immediately started to feel like this new state was permanent that these are all the things I will just have to get used to:

1. I begin to work on accepting that my writer's well has dried up and I'll never write another piece that I like. The book is garbage and I should just throw in the towel.
2. I do an internal sweep of my body to see what's going on. Am I getting sick? Are my lungs rejecting? Do I have an infection at the site of my recent stomach surgery?
3. I feel like my thoughts are dull and uninteresting. Clearly, I've thought my last original thought.
4. Life is generally unsatisfying and surely that won't change.

Then guess what happened? I took a nap. I talked to my friend. I walked my dog. I gave myself permission to take a day or two off from writing. Like a tiny miracle, I felt better. I didn't feel great, but I did feel better.

All of my moods are impermanent, so why am I convinced otherwise? Why am I so ready to accept that my current state is the one I will live in forever? When will I learn to not take my emotions so seriously?

I had this feeling each time I got sick. I get this feeling when I am healthy and I can not imagine ever being sick again. Apparently, based on today, I still have this feeling whenever my moods shift dramatically.

So how does one build a life based on impermanence? Much like building a house on sand—enjoy this moment or tolerate this moment—with no attachment to it being there tomorrow.

Competitive Suffering

I've seen in myself and others who live with serious illness the tendency to compare and judge the severity of another's maladies. Strangely, it can be almost a sense of superiority that underlies the need to pronounce "My boo-boo is bigger than your boo-boo" and write someone off as a big baby or insensitive to the people with *real* problems.

Conversely, I've seen many people who are afraid to share their difficulties with someone like me because they think, "I have no right to complain when I see what other people are dealing with."

The question I pose: Isn't there enough compassion to go around?

One Way Street:

I'm extremely lucky to have wonderful friends who've been with me through thick and thin. They've seen me through dark times of terrible physical and emotional struggles. They've been at my bedside when I was close to death and when I was recovering from transplant surgery. They've seen it all.

I have one friend in particular who, though mostly healthy, has had some of her own health challenges. She's dealt with kidney problems, inexplicable stomach pains and Lyme disease. In addition, she's had some emotionally bumpy times, most notably when her heart was breaking over the end of a seven year relationship.

Despite the "validity" of her hardships, she's often very reluctant to share them with me. She maintains the idea that I've had enough of my own troubles and relaying hers would only be a burden to me. I've repeatedly assured her that I'm her friend and I want to be there for her, the same way she's been there for me. Nonetheless, she can't seem to shake the perception that my problems are bigger than hers and she should just keep them to herself. This makes me very sad.

A Hairy Situation:

After my first transplant, the steroids I was taking beat up my pancreas so much that I became diabetic. This was a whole new frontier for me and I had a few weeks of physical distress while I was learning how to care for this new disease.

I have (had) another friend who's the opposite of the friend I described in the above example. She's usually in crisis mode, more often emotionally than physically. One evening, during this difficult time, she came over to my house unexpectedly. I was having terrible stomach pains and was really unable to talk much. I told her as much and she took that as a cue to talk at me about all of her woes. I think it was about her mother—again. I told her that I was in pain and I started to cry. This new diagnosis had hit me hard and I was worried. She stared at me blankly, let some silent time pass, and resumed her story about her mother. I eventually had to ask her to leave.

This kind of exchange happened many more times. When I was dying the second time, I'd come clean and told her that I thought she was a fair-weather friend. She seemed to disappear during my hard times and come around for advice and comfort when I was feeling better. She apologized and said she understood. We gave our friendship another try.

A few weeks later, I had my second transplant. When I was at home recovering the phone rang. I didn't answer it because I wasn't up to talking to anyone. The message she was leaving on my answering machine was filled with pure panic and horror. I sat bolt upright, and made my way to the phone as soon as possible. Right before I answered it, I heard what she said was causing her so much distress: her hairdresser had colored her hair too dark and she wanted to know what she could do to fix it. That was the last straw for me. I decided I didn't need that kind of inflated hysteria around me anymore and I cut her out of my life.

Compulsive Comparing:

Before transplant, our center requires patients to attend a bi-monthly support group. There we learned about what we would be facing both in the surgery and the recovery. Part of the meeting was to let newly transplanted people tell their stories. Things like, "How long were you on the vent?" and "How many days were you in the hospital?" were high-priority questions. We were all, or so I suspect, inwardly comparing ourselves to the people who had gone before us.

It felt like a lifeline when the patients spoke as if transplant was a piece of cake. Fear pulsed through me when people relayed stories of great difficulty and pain. When people died, it was almost too much to consider.

The obvious truth, however, is that none of those people were me. After all was said and done, none of their experiences matched mine. While they provided me with an anecdotal encyclopedia of possibilities, comparisons were futile and meaningless. When you're embarking on a journey that's so strange and mysterious, it's only human nature to want to apply others' outcomes to your future. Finding a way to take in the story without processing it as your own is very difficult. Difficult, yes, but certainly something to strive for and keep in mind: Compare not!

What I Know Now:

When you have a serious or chronic illness, it can be easy to discount the people around you. To hear someone complain because they have the common cold can seem like an insult. After all, theirs will go away, right? How dare they seek sympathy for something so minor and temporary. If only my greatest problem was a cold!

I must confess, I've had these thoughts and feelings in my life. I've had these feelings and then I got a cold. Wow! Having a cold is miserable! Does the pain I suffer from a broken leg counteract the suffering that comes from a paper cut so that it somehow ceases to be suffering? No. A broken leg is painful and so is a paper cut. They co-exist and are both forms of physical pain. Because one is more severe than the other doesn't cancel out the lesser pain. For me to discount another's suffering based on a comparison to my own is simply a result of self-pity. Ideally, I can have compassion for them as well as for myself.

With that said, there's a sensitivity that's appreciated when one is engaging someone in physical or emotional turmoil. When I'm on a ventilator, please respect my desire for light conversation! When I'm doubled over in pain, please acknowledge my need for peace. When I'm dying, please respect my boundaries and the limits of my energy.

To answer the question I posed above: Yes, there's plenty of compassion to go around. Patients may need to make a conscious effort to give compassion to someone other than themselves. Caregivers may need to make a conscious effort to give themselves permission to acknowledge their own suffering as valid. We all may need to work on being sensitive to each other's personal struggle. And, every once in a while, we may need to part ways because we don't have enough energy to give to each other's wounds. There's compassion in all of these things.

The Illness Identity Crisis

When you become ill, the things that once made up your life begin to fall away. The exercise routines, the jobs, the hobbies—they all pay the price of the body's inability to keep moving. Usually, this causes a crisis of self that I call The Illness Identity Crisis.

Slowly all of the labels we use to define ourselves have been stripped away and we're left with the core of our being. This is a terrifying time when many of us cling to the parts of our life that we have assigned as our identity.

Once the fear dies down, there is an opportunity waiting for you. This is an opportunity to really get to know the untarnished truth of who we really are deep, deep down. Early in my Illness Identity Crisis I was lost and frightened but, eventually, I was able to embrace what it had to offer. I found the beauty of a still body and a forward mind.

Don't You Know Who I Am?

During my time as a medical receptionist, there was one person who we all got to know very well. Her name was June and she had, at one time, been a doctor with a thriving practice. About ten years prior to my meeting her, June had to leave her successful business behind and go on disability. The reasons for this were both emotional and physical. While this was certainly an unfortunate life turn for such a successful person, her story is not what made her stick out in our minds.

June would come in to the office for something small, but would stay for extended periods of time. On some days, she would stand at the front desk for an hour. All the while, the topic of conversation would be the same. Most of her sentences started with "Well, you know I'm a doctor and …" or "When I had my practice we did it this way …"

After establishing her title, she would proceed to ask very trivial questions about the specific suppliers we used for paper, medicine or any other random office staple. She wanted to know if certain suppliers still offered the same discounts as they did when she was practicing and would go into great detail about the price breaks her office enjoyed. If she saw a doctor go by she would inquire with great urgency about types of vaccines being used or about obscure medical treatments she wondered if we had implemented. More often than not, the doctors had no idea what she was talking about. For her final attempt at engaging someone, she would turn to the people in the waiting room and start handing out free advice.

All of this mania was done with her one small item sitting on the counter, yet to be paid for. She kept the reception area hostage while we waited for her payment. In the meantime, she was blocking other clients from checking out or checking in. On more than one occasion, I thought I might explode with irritation. June was out of control.

There is no doubt her behavior was wild and inappropriate. However, when I was able to step back, I saw her exhibitions for what they were: a full blown case of The Illness Identity Crisis. Even after ten years, June had not been able to move forward and redefine herself as something other—or something more—than a doctor. Like a drug addict needing a fix, June came to our office needing to connect with that part of herself that felt powerful. Without another way to identify her value, June was forced to cling to her title as a way to comfort her feelings of loss and purposelessness.

I Am Patient, Hear Me Roar:

There is a flip side to clinging to an old identity. Some people fully embrace their role as patient and assume that as their life's definition. Being waited on, complaining and non-stop conversations about their physical condition become addictive. In certain ways, being sick can make you feel special. The people in your life pay attention to you in ways they wouldn't if you weren't sick. Doctors and other medical professionals are always asking for details on how you are feeling. The world begins to feel as though it revolves around you.

I knew a young man named Daniel who fit this category. He and I were waiting on our lung transplants at the same time. His mother was his biggest fan and no wish of his went unattended. He loved to talk about any and all of his aches and pains—even if they were bathroom issues *nobody* cared to know about. He often expressed his feelings of being cheated and getting the short end of the stick.

Shortly after I had my transplant, Daniel had his. His journey was not a smooth one. The surgery was extremely difficult and his recovery was harder than most. Nonetheless, about a month after his transplant, Daniel went home.

The news of Daniel's post-transplant life was not good. Despite having healthy new lungs, he rarely left the house. His mother reported that he mostly lay on the couch and barked orders at her to get him things. When she refused on the grounds that he was no longer sick, he would throw a tantrum insisting that he was. At one point, he actually confessed to me that he wished he hadn't had the transplant and could go back to the way things were. The team desperately tried to help Daniel adjust to his new reality but, last I saw him, he was still whining and demanding to be waited upon.

This is another form of The Illness Identity Crisis. Defining yourself as a patient can only lead to self-absorption and a desire to stay sick. This is an easy trap to fall into but one that must be consciously avoided.

What's In a Name?:

When you've been given a terminal diagnosis, hopes of "getting better" eventually leave your mind. I was suffering under the weight of all that it meant to die so young. I didn't know what to do or where to go for guidance. There aren't any brochures in the doctor's office on the steps to accepting death at age twenty-nine.

One night I was sitting in front of a glass door. I was crying and looking out into the dark night. At one point, my vision shifted and I was no longer looking outside but at the image of myself reflecting back at me. There I was, Tiffany, a young woman with red hair in a green shirt crying and thinking about death. My image was translucent and I could see through it to the trees behind the door.

As my eyes moved back and forth, I saw meaning in this reflection. This girl, the one with red hair and a green shirt, was temporary, so temporary she was merely an illusion. Tiffany was the name given to her, but Tiffany in no way described her entirety. This reflection was a perfect representation of the reality of my existence. I was able to see my physical presence and my eternal self all in one.

It was that night that I was able to say goodbye. Goodbye to the physical image, the red hair, green shirt and the name Tiffany. I was also able to embrace the part of that image I wasn't able to see with my eyes but feel with my insides—the permanent, translucent part of me that has no name or hair color. "Tiffany" is only a part of me. There's so much more to who I am than what I can see. With that exercise, I was able to let go of the parts of my identity that were only temporary.

Internal Playground:

Purpose. Isn't that what most of us are looking for? When I was waiting for my first transplant, the lack of purpose in my life was so profound I could barely stand it. I felt worthless without that all-important job, relationship or overall reason to get up in the morning. It didn't matter to me that I was dying and waiting for a lung transplant. That didn't take me off the mental hook and I felt like I needed to be *doing* something.

That's when I turned inwards. I didn't have the physical strength to "work" in an outward way, so I created a job for my inner self. I thought about myself and what I liked and didn't like. I thought about what I'd most like to improve upon. I decided I needed to learn how to be a more compassionate person. I called my job Project Compassion, and dedicated myself to reading about, praying about and practicing compassion. Soon, my inner life began to open up in ways I never knew possible. I was connected to myself, a higher power and others in a way I hadn't ever been before. I created a world within myself that was stimulating, satisfying and gave me a clear sense of purpose.

My core is an indescribable, un-namable part of my being with no adjectives or duties associated with it. There's great healing in knowing who you are without any labels. My core was never sick or tired or even scared. By exploring new landscapes with me, I was able to connect with a much deeper sense of who I am. While I no longer had many external labels, I began to have new definitions for my identity. I discovered who I was at the very core of my being.

What I Know Now:

When the body can't function at its optimal speed and ability it can be very frustrating, or even depressing. It can be the beginning of a long journey to discovering who you are without all the worldly trappings. I hope perhaps you'll now see this time as an opportunity to discover places within yourself that few people have the time or inclination to explore within themselves. It won't stop being hard, but it can be a time of great purpose and learning. Invite the Illness Identity Crisis and see all the riches it has to offer. This applies to those with serious and chronic illness as well as those staying home for a week with the flu!

On Being Judgmental

Journal entry from July, 2003

I've been noticing lately how much I really enjoy judging people in my head. If I can find a way to make their behavior seem illogical or reckless, I can delight in climbing up on my high horse and pronouncing them less than I. It makes me feel powerful. I've had a few instances recently that gave me some new insights into the root of my judgmental behavior.

At dinner the other night, my brother-in-law, Jack, was talking about a cough he'd been dealing with for the past week or so. I became angry and scolded him for not going to the doctor. I spoke to him sarcastically and attempted to shame him for being irresponsible with his health. Jack doesn't respond to this kind of outburst and my attitude was dismissed, next topic.

Later, I felt embarrassed by my behavior. Why had I reacted so strongly to reports of a simple cough? At first, I assumed it was a reaction born out of self-pity. How could he so casually ignore a cough when lung problems had been my greatest downfall? Why did he get to be so leisurely about it when I had to take it so seriously?

While I'm sure there were elements of truth to that theory, it didn't ring true as a whole. I dug a little deeper into the subtext of the exchange and uncovered my underlying emotions were not anger or self-pity; they were fear and worry.

Years ago, when I was in ICU following my first lung transplant, Jack was very ill at home with pneumonia. It had started with a cough that he didn't address and the consequence was a yucky bout of pneumonia. My anger and sarcasm were a manifestation of my fear that he would, once again, neglect himself and wind up very sick.

So why the anger? Why did that emerge instead of the love that provided a foundation for my worry? Why would I choose, consciously or unconsciously, to address him in that way instead of with kindness? The answer: vulnerability.

Kindness makes me feel vulnerable, judgment makes me feel strong. Clearly, these feelings don't benefit anyone and are simply counter-productive. Kindness or concern would have gone over much better than misplaced anger and criticism. Perhaps that same exchange delivered with heartfelt concern would have brought us closer together. Instead the opposite was true.

I've taken this realization and attempted to apply it to my life. The results have been interesting.

I was getting frustrated with my boyfriend the other day. Out of all of the people in my life, Pete was the only one who hadn't made a "happy painting" for our kitchen wall. He'd promised to do one over and over but never delivered. I just didn't understand what the problem was. I began to pester him about this, again, and his reaction was to get defensive. I stopped myself in mid-sentence and decided to try and tap into the deeper reason behind my irritation.

Once I took a moment to do this, I was able to see that my reasons for wanting him to create a painting reflected my desire for him to let go of his chronic fear of failure. I knew Pete was putting off the painting because of his overwhelming fear that the painting wouldn't be good enough, deep enough, clever enough—not because he didn't want to do one. This precise fear held him back from many other life experiences. He had a history of quitting before he began.

From where I was sitting, in the land of carpe diem, this kind of resistance to life's new territories was tragic. I wanted so badly for him to break through that mentality and my conscious manifestation of that desire was to judge him for his perceived cowardice. When I was able to get in touch with this deeper emotion, as well as the shallowness of my judgment, I stopped my ranting.

Instead, I sat down next to him, looked him in the eye and told him the truth from my heart. I told him I wanted him to do this painting because he was such an important person in my life; the wall would simply not be complete without his contribution. I told him I didn't care if the painting was a Mona Lisa or pure nonsense, I just wanted him to have the experience of painting on canvas. I told him I loved him and wanted him to feel safe to try something new. The honesty that poured from me made both of us well up with tears. It was a kind of shift in a moment that I'd never experienced before. It was beautiful, real and freeing.

Pete never made a painting but I never brought it up again. It no longer bothered me and I certainly felt no need to nag him about it. I had spoken my true feelings and the rest was up to him. I was fine with whatever he chose and had no judgments.

There's something easy and satisfying about judging and gossiping. If there weren't, so many of us wouldn't be reading celebrity magazines! I can't pretend that these discoveries have transformed me to a place of non-judgmental nirvana. The difference is that I now know when I'm doing it and that a much more satisfying alternative exists. It's in my hands to stop taking the easy way out and do a little extra work in order to find a much kinder and more rewarding way to engage those I love.

The Pain of Positive Thinking

At some point in a person's life, they usually stumble upon the allure of the power of positive thinking. In our culture it seems to be gaining popularity as a way to combat illness. Apparently, if I believe I am healthy, I will be. If I believe I am rich I will be. Once I know the secrets of how to think my way to success, I will have anything I desire.

While the concept of positive thinking is certainly valuable and useful, taken to extremes it can also be very destructive.

If You Believe, It Still May Not Be So:

When I was in my mid-twenties I moved to California and became deeply immersed in my spirituality. Part of that included a mentorship with a well-known female guru I'll call Tisha. She had a rather large following and I was always honored when I was able to get face time with her alone. I respected her tremendously and was an eager student.

I was being trained that nothing in this world is a coincidence, that we have control of our own lives. I learned how to pray for things and they would happen. I learned to value myself as an important child of God. I worked hard to believe in myself and in my future.

The one thing that I wasn't able to "transform" was my health. I'd still get sick and continued coming and going from in-patient hospital care.

Tisha told me I could be well if only I wanted it enough and believed that it could happen. At first this was an inspiring concept and one I embraced fully. I visualized my healing and trusted God would provide me with a way out of my physical ailments. Time passed and my health continued to deteriorate despite my prayers and affirmations. Tisha's words rang in my ears: "You can be well if you only want it enough and believe it can be so." I *thought* I wanted it. I *thought* I believed it could be so. I assumed I merely hadn't dug deep enough and had hidden resistance to health in my unconscious self.

My failure to heal slowly led to a failure to believe in my own spiritual depth. I told myself that if I only prayed harder, loved God more or believed more strongly, I'd be free of this disease. I pleaded with God to show me how to dig deep enough to heal my mutated genes. I began to feel bad about myself and thought of myself as a miserable failure. I beat myself up for my perceived inadequacies.

Eventually, I became depressed. By believing that I had the power to change my illness, I had to accept the opposite as true: *remaining sick was my fault.* I took full responsibility for the continued decline of my health. All the while, my disease kept on progressing without a hint of it recognizing my spiritual journey.

Form:

Before my first transplant, I had a great teacher in acting school. He was from Russia and taught an exciting movement class. He taught us a movement ritual, that he called Form, every day. When he would hear me coughing he'd assure me that if I just did Form enough, I'd be cured. I thought he was out of his mind but secretly tried it anyway. He was wrong.

What I Know Now:

So many people have the magic bullet, that thing they know about that will fix any problem. From self-help gurus to nutritionists to spiritual teachers, they all boast the right recommendations and advice. There's nothing wrong with embracing these ideas. When it becomes a problem is when you don't allow the possibility for them not to solve everything.

What I've come to realize is that we're all made of matter and are earthbound creatures. Because of this, we must abide by the rules of *earth*. Sometimes miracles happen. Often, they don't. The stories people tell are those of the miracles. The stories of the people who fought and prayed and believed and *died anyway* are the stories that don't get put into books or the movie of the week.

Are we so dense as to only understand a miracle to be an unexplained cure?

What about the miracle of loving life despite illness?

Why isn't it ever considered part of the plan for a person to be sick?

There is great potential for pain and heartache within the teachings of Positive Thinking. There's certainly nothing wrong with working for better health, that is, unless you'll define yourself as a failure if it doesn't come true. Many of today's "thinking into being" schools take an extremely simplistic approach to healing. This is irresponsible and detrimental. Feed your spirit with love and compassion but beware of the Pain of Positive Thinking.

Tiffany's Top Ten Opportunities of Illness

1. Getting the chance to say goodbye

2. Learning to stand up for what you need, even in the face of "authority"

3. Learning compassion for yourself and others

4. Using limitations as a motivation to try something you would have never thought to try

5. Learning how to be In the Moment

6. Getting the chance to learn who you *really* are, without all the frills

7. The chance to resolve differences with those you love

8. Discovering what you *really* think about God and where we go next

9. Going to an internal place that is so deep pain can not find you there

10. Finding gratitude—truly appreciating, perhaps for the first time, all the sights, smells, tastes and feelings that earth has to offer

Healing vs. Medicating

At one point during my illness career, my best friend dragged me to a four night conference to listen to a Buddhist Lama. I'd just lost a good transplant buddy and was feeling sorry for his death and my own physical crosses to bear.

If you've ever heard a Buddhist Lama speak, you know they tend to say the same thing over and over again. It may sound boring, but it's usually is quite powerful. The Lama began by repeating the phrase "Happiness comes from the inside." I nodded my head in complete agreement. Here in the west, we've accepted that money, fame and material possessions can't fulfill a human heart. Of course, despite this, we still spend plenty of time and energy striving for those exact things. "Happiness comes from the inside." Yes, I was in complete agreement that my own happiness comes from my love of life, myself and the divine. "Happiness comes from the inside." Certainly, yes!

Suddenly, however, the phrase changed and my head was no longer nodding in agreement. "Suffering comes from the inside." What? How could he say such a thing? Does that mean I've chosen to suffer the difficulty and pain of all of my body's maladies? "Suffering comes from the inside." How dare he suggest that my suffering is something I could control! My suffering comes from a physical ailment that was given to me by a genetic twist of the DNA. "Suffering comes from the inside." What an insult to me and those I love who have dealt with serious illness. No!

It took me a few weeks to understand what he was talking about. He was talking about the difference between healing and medicating.

Brush with Death:

I was dying again. I had chronic rejection, with very little hope of another transplant, and I spent most of my time alone at home. The doctors had told me there was little they could do to help me. The television became my greatest companion. I had a detailed program schedule I would adhere to every day. As one might imagine, this routine became empty and lonely.

I decided it was time to find a project to keep me busy. The challenge, of course, was finding something I was physically able to do. I tried to think of things that a person could do while remaining nearly still as well as something I had never done before. With these criteria as my guide, I elected to try my hand at painting—despite a complete lack of artistic talent and training.

I started with a small canvas and a few paints. I found that with little physical effort I could sit and create something from nothing. I was hooked. My canvases got bigger and bigger, and it was the highlight of my day. I looked forward to the times when I had the energy to paint. When I wasn't painting, I was often thinking about painting. I felt alive when I was creating. When I was painting, my joy overcame my suffering.

I was so infected with the joy of painting I required it of my visitors as well. I bought many mini-canvases and asked all of my guests—people tend to visit you when you're dying—to paint something that made them happy. Most people complied and it was so much fun to see what each individual would come up with! Soon, my kitchen walls were covered with paintings from those I love. It was very special.

As I grew gravely ill, I was no longer able to paint for more than a few minutes. I was working on a massive canvas with small mosaic-like blue squares. When people noticed that I wasn't going to finish, they took up where I left off. That painting is hanging above my couch now and is called Group Effort. It's, by far, my favorite painting of all time.

None of my artworks were masterpieces—or even moderately attractive—but that wasn't the point. With a failing body, I was able to find excitement and creativity within myself that I didn't know was still there. When I was painting I wasn't aware of my illness. During a time when there were no more medicines to help me, I was healing through joy. To be clear, painting did not heal my body, but it certainly was medicine for my soul.

What I Know Now:

Healing is something that can be done no matter what the physical diagnosis. When we bow to the skills of our medical team, we think that we're asking for healing. In fact, what they have to offer us is merely medicating. Ideally, we would incorporate both into our lives. Let the trained professionals do the poking, prescribing and cutting. It's the patient's job to do the healing.

Many people pray for, and some experience, miracles of unexplainable recovery from illness. What I learned is that there's another kind of miracle that's not nearly so dramatic. That's the miracle of learning to love life despite serious disability or terminal illness.

I may have been trapped in a body that wasn't going to be cured by a miracle, but it was up to me to decide if I wanted to stay trapped in my self-made prison, or to escape the bars through by learning the lessons this broken-down old body had to teach me.

In time, I learned that the illness wasn't my choice, but whether or not to suffer was. Every day, I had the choice to focus on my physical pains or my inner joy. What I never understood before going to hear the Lama speak was that the two can simultaneously exist.

If I were listening to the same Lama today, I'd surely be nodding my head in agreement. "Happiness comes from the inside. Suffering comes from the inside." Certainly, yes!

God Isn't a Magician

Journal entry from April, 2001

It has suddenly occurred to me that God isn't the God I imagined as a child and have deeply embedded in my subconscious. God isn't the controlling miracle worker. God can't make me go to sleep when I'm not tired. God can't heal my lungs when they're sick. God can't create money for me when I'm poor. God doesn't do magic tricks.

God is merely and profoundly my guide. God wills me to relax my thoughts so I might go to sleep. God guides me to good doctors, and away from bad ones, so I might be educated about a healthy way of life and given good medicine. God leads me to people who can give me a job so I can make the money I need. God doesn't do magic tricks. God simply leads me and I have the choice of whether or not to listen.

It's up to me whether or not I let my mind calm down, take the doctor's advice, or accept the job that will provide some money. I'm ultimately the one who makes the choice to sleep, be healthy or healthier, and to have money.

I was raised believing God could do anything, and now I know he can't do anything without my cooperation. Cooperation comes in the form of integrity and openness. If I'm without integrity, I will make the negative choice. If I'm not open, I can't be guided by the spirits' gentle whispers.

I must stop sleeping through life. I must start taking more time to allow the opportunity for spirit to speak to me. I must give my own spirit the respect it deserves for being responsible for ending up where I am. I must accept that responsibility for every shape, every nuance of my life. I must listen at every step.

God isn't a magician and if I fall out of the boat, he can't wave his wand and zap me back in.

The Vulnerability of Illness

In so many ways, illness challenges us to question who we are. Often, it takes away parts of our identity and leaves us wondering what's left. As if that isn't enough, we find ourselves being handled by strangers and stripped of our independence. Despite our age, we all must struggle with the kind of helplessness that usually comes to us in childhood. Like a passenger on a runaway train, we have no access to the brakes and can only pray that the ones in charge will take good care of us. It's quite a disturbing place to be.

My Life in His Hands:

The day after my first transplant, a team of physical therapists descended upon me and took me for a walk around the halls of ICU. I was still on the ventilator so they had to disconnect me from the machine. As a replacement, they attached the tube in my lungs to a bag. One of the techs had to squeeze it to breathe for me. I was miserable and very freaked out. With each squeeze of the bag came another surge of anxiety. The techs were happily chatting about their weekend or some other non-medical topic. What if the one breathing for me lost focus and missed a squeeze? What if he got off rhythm? I couldn't talk and it was all I could do to take the next step. My most basic bodily instinct, breathing, was being controlled by someone whom I'd just met and who didn't seem to take this responsibility very seriously. I was at his mercy in a way I'd never been before and couldn't have imagined. Of course, he did his job and I was returned to my bed unharmed. Nonetheless, I was thrilled to be reconnected to the machine. It seemed much more reliable and made me feel far less vulnerable.

On Display:

I was filled with tubes. I had IVs in my neck, a tube draining my urine and what felt like a fire hose coming out of my nose. My mother and my husband were by my side as I underwent my first big contrast study after the Nissen fun-doplication. When the test was done, they offered to wheel me to my room in order to avoid the long wait for transport.

The test had been done in the basement of the hospital, many floors and a few wings away from the safety of my private room. Getting back proved to be a challenge.

My husband was pushing the wheelchair and my mother manned the IV pole. Sometimes, the long IV tubes would get caught in the wheelchair. It was a much more difficult endeavor than either one had anticipated. With caution they made their way through the hospital and we ended up in the familiar territory of the main hospital lobby. This lobby stretches along the entire front of the building and leads to the elevators that would take us back to my room.

I had never noticed it until that day, but not many in-patients are in that lobby. I was the only one I saw in a gown. I was certainly the only one with a fire hose taped to my nose. I became acutely aware that my urine was on display. I felt terribly embarrassed. I put my head down and braced myself until we had cleared all of the many fixated eyeballs. On that journey, I understood the value of the professional transport system: they would have gone the back way.

Later, I told my husband how the trip through the lobby made me feel. He had no idea I was feeling that way and he felt horrible about it. I knew he hadn't intended to embarrass me but he apologized anyway. I think this experience was a tremendous learning opportunity for him. I know he will look at things a little differently given a similar situation in the future.

What I Know Now:

There's a big difference between emotional vulnerability and physical vulnerability. I can choose to let someone see my deepest feelings, share my most painful experiences, and I can choose to stop the sharing at any time. In a similar way, I can choose to be physically vulnerable but would only do that with someone I love, trust and want to have that kind of intimacy with. However, when I'm lying in a hospital bed and I'm being touched and moved and wiped—I'm sorry, but that's reality—I can't imagine being able to let myself feel okay about that physical vulnerability. It's more like an assault than the voluntary giving you share with someone you love.

It helps if the caregiver is the same sex. It definitely helps if they're very sensitive to what's happening. Honestly, though, I have a very hard time imagining a situation in which it could ever feel empowering.

As a sick person, you can feel like you spend your life at the mercy of others; waiting for them to bring you food, medicine, oxygen; being pushed in a wheelchair at a speed and route not determined by you. Being sick feels like being out of control.

Caregivers can make a big difference in how vulnerable someone in that position feels. Simply by being gentle and respectful with their body can make a huge difference. You can never underestimate the value of your kind words, or lack thereof. In small moments that are simply routine parts of life with illness, you have so much power to change the way a patient feels.

As a patient, you'll have to find the balance between organizing your care in a way that allows you to retain some control, and accept there will be times in which you'll have to hand the reins over to someone else. For the times that you find yourself at the mercy of others, you'll need to find a way to breath through the discomfort.

There's no easy solution to this problem. Vulnerability is one of the most emotionally painful parts of illness. Perhaps accepting this as part of the illness package is the only defense there is.

That Which Is Important

Journal entry from March, 2007

It's been years since my second transplant. I've worked so hard to rejoin society! I have a "real" job now and 2.5 children. Two dogs and a bird count, right? I pay my own bills and have a wonderful husband. I live in a nice home, rented, but nice. I have some friends and a few hobbies. I'm working on my dream to be a (paid) public speaker. From where I sit, I'm doing everything there's to do to hold my place as a "normal" member of this society. I'm living the rat race and the dream all at once.

With all of this, I've lost hold of one of illness's greatest gifts; the clarity, in day-to-day living, of That Which Is Important. Lately, I've been focusing on this and trying to bring it back. I've been amazed at how unsuccessful I've been.

That Which Is Important is all that's sacred and sweet about life. It's enjoying all that this physical plane, this earth, has to offer. Jacob and I hold hands as a natural display of affection and connectedness. How many times do I hold his hand and really feel the texture of his skin, the gentleness of his grip? Very rarely. This is usually something that I do absent mindedly. Today, I put all of my consciousness into the grasp of his hand and I was overwhelmed with tenderness. The touch of his skin was intoxicating and I felt like the luckiest person in the world to have the opportunity to hold such a perfect hand. This is what it's like to be in touch with That Which Is Important.

I was able to catch a few more fleeting glimpses today when I ate my favorite Mexican meal, cuddled my silly dog and had a good laugh about the possum on our front porch. It's a matter of simultaneously being in the moment and being just outside of it enough to appreciate its simple magnificence. It's a moment of profoundly deep gratitude.

When I was very sick, this kind of connection with That Which Is Important was very natural. It was as though there was a grid in front of me and I could see the connection between events and individuals so clearly. I could easily see how we, as humans, stand in our own way with self-doubt and complicated excuses. I watched people miss the beauty in their own struggles. Things just made sense. Since I've crashed back to earth with my physical health, this grid has disappeared. I'm once again, standing on the ground with two feet, confused and full of self doubt.

I imagine when we leave this earth certain kinds of experiences won't be available to us. No longer in a physical form, food and touch (and possums?) won't be a part of existence. For this reason, it's imperative that I stay aware of all of the modest parts of living that, when noticed, are truly exquisite. In this whirlwind of a world, I will continue the struggle to remember That Which Is Important.

Family Support Dynamics

When someone is very ill, family dynamics can be delicate. There are burdens placed on family members and resentment can brew if the weight isn't evenly distributed. The problem is, not everyone is equipped to be the down-and-dirty caregiver. Not everyone lives in the same town or state as the patient. Reality dictates that an even distribution is just not going to happen.

No matter the situation, I've found that every family member brings their unique skills and gifts to the table. If these skills and gifts are recognized, they can be an integral part of the support network, even if part of that network can't stand needles.

Love Doesn't Require Fainting:

Luckily for me, my mother can handle needles, blood and other unpleasant bodily by-products. My father, on the other hand, tried to be in the room a few times when I was getting an IV and he nearly fainted each time. He doesn't have the constitution to be the person who'll hold my hand when things are being pulled out or poked or cleaned up. There was a time when that might have made him feel bad, but, at some point it became clear that there were other things he could do that made a big difference.

My father has always handled the headache of insurance and hospital paperwork. When I was sick, I never had to deal with the annoyance of getting things approved or sorting out the complicated payment issues. I'm forever grateful for that.

Dad also did a great job of pitching in when he could to make life easier on Mom and me. I often had to do IV therapy at home, and a few of the drugs had to be mixed up less than one hour before the dose was given. This was very aggravating, especially in the middle of the night! Nonetheless, my father took this on as his job and I never had to worry about mixing up my meds again. They were always waiting for me when the time came. What a relief.

My father did a good portion of the spoiling too. My appetite was often very poor so when I had a craving for something it was an event to celebrate. Unfortunately, those cravings didn't always happen at convenient times. My dad was always willing to run out, no matter what time, and track down the food I desired. I remember one time when he actually convinced my favorite Italian place to make me a pizza after they'd closed! His willingness to do this made me feel very loved.

Dad avoids direct contact with all things medically painful or physically distressing. Better that than to scrape him off the floor! Mom holds my hand during all the procedures while Dad does many other valuable things to support me in my times of need.

Morphine and Sign Language:

Sometimes the contribution a person makes to a difficult situation is entirely unpredictable. My two sisters and their families live nearby and have seen me weekly through all my highs and lows. My brother, on the other hand, lives far away and we only get to visit a few times a year. Despite the distance, he turned out to be extraordinarily helpful after both of my transplants.

Jim flew down and was by my side, with the rest of my wonderful family, the day after both surgeries. During that time I was intubated and couldn't speak. This was an especially distressing time for me as I had many questions and comments that I could not voice. I attempted my version of sign language— more like a morphine-inhibited game of charades—but nobody could understand me. Except Jim.

I don't know what it was or how he knew but he always comprehended my silly hand signals. Whenever I started trying to communicate, people learned to go get Jim. It was so soothing to know there was someone who could answer my questions and even get my hand-signal jokes!

There was no way to predict Jim was going to be so helpful in that capacity but it was very sweet that he was. It made me feel so much closer to my brother, and I'll never forget all of our mute conversations; no matter how hazy the drugs were making me feel!

What I Know Now:

Support can come in many forms. Taking care of a sick loved one requires a team. It's easy to place expectations on people that don't match with what they're able to do well and comfortably. Families and patients should keep on the look-out for what an individual naturally gravitates towards. Would you rather run errands than spend long hours sitting by the bedside? Would you rather have long heart-to-hearts about life and death in lieu of dealing with the insurance company? Everyone has a part to play. The trick is figuring out who does what, and honoring each other's roles as equally valuable.

A Prayer for Mom and Dad

Journal entry from Christmas, 2003

One of the hardest parts of illness is the helplessness that comes with being taken care of by loved ones. In a dark time, this helplessness can manifest itself as resentment. In an enlightened time, this helplessness manifests as an overwhelming gratitude for a debt so huge it could never be repaid. This gratitude easily transforms into guilt.

The only way I've been able to let go of my guilt is to stop believing that it's within my power to repay and reward those I love for all they've done for me. I wrote this poem/prayer in a moment of hopeless guilt as a way to free myself of the weight of my gratitude.

To my beautiful parents
Who have nursed me when I was sick,
Let me run when I was well,
And sat by my side as we cried both
tears of laughter and of sadness.

There's nothing I could ever do on this
earth to repay all the sacrifices you've
made or the love you have given me
throughout the years, so all I can offer
is this prayer:

I pray that, whether in this world or the
next, all the generosity you have shown
me will bring a smile to God's eyes and
he will reward you in ways you never
imagined.

Amen

In the Bed vs. By the Bed

I've always felt that I'd rather be in the bed than be the one standing by the bed. It seems like it would be so scary and there would be such an immense feeling of powerlessness. I've only had minimal experiences as a caregiver but have worked for hospice and studied them a little bit. As always, my views on this topic come mostly from the patient perspective.

Family Feud:

I was called to a hospice situation one day to provide respite for the family. I was met at the main house by a very weird attitude—not unkind, just not the usual warmth and grief. I was told that my patient was in the guest house and that I should go over there instead. I walked there unescorted and was promptly greeted by two women. Before I could finish introducing myself and enquiring about the patient, they'd already launched into the family drama that surrounded my patient.

Apparently, the woman in the first house was their sister/aunt and they hated her. The mother-daughter team were visiting from the west coast to see Mom/Grandma for the last time. The real reason I was called there was to make sure that The Duo could leave and The Sister could enter without actually having to see each other. I was there to provide air traffic control.

I was introduced to the barely conscious patient. She was on a lot of morphine and had no interest in me. I sat by her bed and made sure she was okay while The Sister and The Duo traded places. About five minutes after the mother and daughter left, Sister entered with two of her children who were somewhere between six and ten.

Sister visited with her mom and proceeded to force her child to kiss Grandma. The child was scared and Grandma was unconscious. Eventually my patient woke up and Sister immediately held her hand and began to tell her that she and The Duo were still fighting and that they would never get along.

Mom whispered, "I love you" and fell back to sleep.

147

Sister and her children soon left, and I sat with the sleeping patient for another half hour or so. The phone rang and I answered, as instructed. It was The Duo and they were ready to come back. They needed to know if the coast was clear. I told them it was and they said they were on their way. They called two more times on the way back from town to make one hundred percent sure that Sister really wasn't there anymore.

As soon as they crossed over the threshold, they resumed Sister-bashing. I stood listening for about ten more minutes before I told them I needed to leave. They asked how Mom was and wanted to talk more about Sister. I again excused myself and almost ran to the car.

I cried all the way home and felt sick for another few days. If I had to pick one thing to have when I'm dying, it would be peace. Peace in my home, peace in my relationships and peace in my heart. That poor woman was days away from death and her children still wanted her to play the role of mediator and mother. Her job was done and it was their turn to provide the nurturing. They couldn't see past their own agendas to give their mother that precious gift.

My patient died two days after my visit. I wish her eternal peace and I wish her family healing.

Care for Two:

I have a lot of pride. I don't like to wear hospital gowns, I don't like to be nurse-handled and I don't like pity. Before my transplants, long stays in the hospital were routine. I'd go in with horrible lung infections and be given powerful IV antibiotics for weeks. I'm not sure which makes you feel worse, the infection or the antibiotics. There were many times when I felt too weak and too sick to take a shower. My mother would offer to wash my hair and I'd always refuse. It just felt too vulnerable and my pride prevailed over the griminess I was feeling.

One day I guess I'd reached my limit and I told my mom I wanted to wash my hair somehow, someway. She sprung into action and began putting together an elaborate system of buckets, pitchers and pillows. I positioned myself at the end of the bed and she poured water over my hair and it fell into the bucket below. She scrubbed my hair and it was as if I'd been reborn! Never underestimate a clean head of hair!

Over the years, we have perfected this technique and do it often—we now use a chair tilted by the shower. The lesson learned, other than the healing powers of shampoo, is that this kind of activity is equally helpful for both parties. I got the obvious benefits but it was clear to me that my mother benefited too. She got to do something to make her daughter feel better. Those kinds of opportunities weren't common. It brought us closer together, and I'm so thankful I pushed my pride aside so I could let her help me. Sometimes it's the nicest thing a patient can do for the ones caring for them.

What I Know Now:

When you're sick, it's very easy to fall into the pattern of constantly focusing on yourself and your current state. Being a caregiver is a very stressful and sometimes horrible position to be in. Remember to be aware that your caregivers have difficulties too. Remember they can burn out and need some balance, a.k.a. get away from you. Don't forget to look outside yourself and see all that they do for you, then share your gratitude.

Most importantly, be honest with yourself. Could you get up and get that drink of water yourself but you've just fallen into the habit of asking for things? Is your current complaint bad enough that you need to share it? If not, there's nothing wrong with keeping it to yourself. Have you asked your loved one how *they're* doing today?

There's a fine balance between getting the support you need and becoming an overwhelming, all-consuming drain on those you love. Do for yourself when you can, respectfully ask for something when you can't. There'll certainly be times of stress and crisis when being polite may fly out the window, but remaining conscious of how hard those around you're working—emotionally and physically—can only be beneficial to everyone involved.

The Death Bed Myth

Journal entry from September, 2003

I suppose I've seen lots of movies in which one of the characters is dying. I'm not really sure where I formed my unconscious fantasies about the way things would be when I was on my death bed. All I know for sure is that I had a belief that when I was dying, things would change. I believed that:

The world would slow down, maybe even stop.
I'd be surrounded by loved ones at all times.
Relationship conflicts would miraculously resolve.
There would be many deep confessions, laughter and tears.
Worldly things would cease—bills, toilet malfunctions, dirty dishes.
I'd know I was dying.

It's a shock to discover that my vision of what lay ahead was more a mirage than a reality. I've been very surprised to find that:

The world keeps spinning at the same speed.
People still go to work and live their lives.
Difficult relationships are still difficult and actually can become more so.
You feel a great amount of ambiguity around death. When exactly does being really sick cross over to dying? They feel very much the same!

News Flash! Dying isn't as glamorous as they make it look on soap operas. I didn't even know I had expectations of what it would be like to die. Now, I feel great disappointment in knowing that my unconscious expectations had it all wrong.

Equal Opportunity Compassion

There's a well-known truth that illness doesn't only affect the individual who's afflicted but has a profound impact on their family and friends as well. The sicker I got, the more pronounced the reactions of the people around me. Often I was surprised and occasionally I was disappointed by those I loved. What I eventually came to see was that the way they treated me rarely had much to do with me at all. Illness and dying are not areas of comfort for most people. Some people were able to transcend their discomfort and reach out; others retreated, unable to bypass their own fears.

Go With the Flow:

When I was very sick and was believed to be dying, I had family members and friends who came forward in ways that were truly remarkable. I can't tell you if they were scared or uncomfortable because, if they were, they didn't show it. They met me where I was and engaged me in conversations about saying good-bye and how I wanted to be remembered.

One friend in particular drove from another town to visit me once a week. She didn't arrive with expectations being entertained or of even having a good talk. She brought things to occupy herself, like sewing materials or knitting. She'd sit with me in the living room and let me lead the day.

Sometimes we would talk at length about life and death. Sometimes we would laugh about superficial, silly things. Sometimes we barely spoke at all and I'd watch TV and nap while she read her book or worked on her latest craft project. I always looked forward to her visit and found her willingness to sit with whatever came up to be brave and admirable.

Punished and Pitied:

There were people in my life who carried with them a thick lens focused only on their own reality. It was difficult for them to see beyond that lens, and, at times, this made me feel uncomfortable and judged. I had one relative in particular who approached me with great pity in his eyes. He told me that when he saw me, so sickly and frail, his reaction was to wonder why God had let such a thing happen to me. Why was I being punished so?

I attempted to explain to him that I didn't feel punished. In fact, I felt the opposite. I felt connected to the universe and at peace. The pity in his eyes didn't wash away, no matter how much I told him of my experience. Our very different perspectives made it difficult for me to be around him and I certainly could no longer look him in the eye.

Loved and Left:

There were people in my life who couldn't overcome their own discomfort with illness and dying. They were at one time very close to me, but, as I got sicker, they withdrew from my life more and more. At first, I felt angry and abandoned by their retreat. I tried to engage them in conversation about how I felt about my current state of dying and they rarely responded. I was in a unique world of suffering and fascination and couldn't understand why they would ignore me at such a pivotal time.

Eventually, I grew to understand their fears outweighed their love. It hurt too much to be around me. They hadn't yet accepted their own mortality and therefore were unable to accept mine.

Bold, Bewildering and Beautiful:

When I was dying, someone close to me made an unusual offer. He saw I was suffering, and he told me, if I ever got to the point where I couldn't take it anymore, he'd be willing to help me by finding someone who would euthanize me. I'd never even considered the possibility.

"No thanks!" I cried, shocked and taken aback. Despite my physical discomforts, my internal spiritual world was so exciting I didn't dare cut it short. I'd some day reach the end of this life, and I was invested in seeing how it would play out.

Later, when I was able to think about his proposal, I could see that he made a bold and brave move out of love for me. I imagine he fears that part of life, the pain and suffering that comes with dying. Because he loved me, he wanted to offer me what he'd want someone to offer him: a way out. It took guts for him to offer me something that many people would want but would never dare to vocalize. I thank him for his compassion.

What I Know Now:

Today, I have a very different outlook than I did at the time. There's no way to predict how those you love might react to an illness. What I discovered was that I had a certain expectation of how I should be treated and that expectation was rarely the reality. Looking back, I can see my expectations were also entirely unfair. To expect everyone to be at ease in such a hard circumstance is unreasonable. To expect people to act exactly the way you would like them to is absurd.

I expected compassion from those in my life, but what I failed to do was also *give* compassion. I placed myself in the center of the universe and forgot that others had deep feelings of their own. I felt entitled to some particular kind of attention, and, when I didn't get it, I allowed myself to feel victimized.

Some people will step forward. Some people will step back. Some people will judge. What was hard for me to see was that all of those actions are results of love. Just as those facing illness must receive love and compassion, so must those dealing with people facing illness. Just because you're sick, doesn't mean you can't be the one to reach out to another.

While it was easier to see the gifts brought by those willing to sit with me in my tiny illness cocoon, I now see the value of the lessons brought by those unable to do so. I'm grateful to all the people in my life, no matter how their love chose to manifest itself.

Saying Goodbye to Those You Love

Journal entry from August, 2003

I've heard stories about people who died of an illness and their family never even knew they were sick. They hid their medical prognosis and died alone. How could someone not let their family know they were dying? Why would they be so secretive? Were they cowards or martyrs? I never understood this.

I never understood—until now. Doctor Newland told me weeks ago that I only had six months to live and I still haven't told my family. I just got back from a week at the beach; everyone was there. I didn't have any fun and I was being a real bitch because all I could think about was whether or not to take this opportunity to reveal my news and ruin their vacation. Ultimately, I left without saying anything. A few miles from the beach house, I pulled over to the side of the road and contemplated going back to make my announcement. I just couldn't do it. I left the beach and cried most of the way home.

When's the right time to tell all of the people you love that this is the end of the line? What day is a good day for learning this information? A weekend, perhaps, so you can process before you go back to work? But I've just ruined their weekend. Should I tell them individually or as a group? Would it be okay to just keep this information to myself? Would that be wrong?

This is, by far, the hardest thing I've ever had to do. I wish I could just run away and die alone. I get it now, I really do.

Like Most Girls:
A Love Story

Like most young girls, I spent hours dreaming of the day I'd meet a man and fall in love. Romantic dates, wedding dresses, and images of happily-ever-after danced through my head. All the while, the nagging question underneath: "But can a girl who's so sick have all those things?"

Dating isn't easy for anyone. Proof of that can be found simply by visiting the self-help section of any bookstore! Whether we're trying to figure out the "rules" of dating or understand the differences between Mars and Venus, there clearly are a lot of people in need of guidance on the topic. Most of us reach a point in our lives when we deeply desire a partner and rarely have a smooth journey in finding, or, for that matter, keeping one.

Acknowledging the already challenging nature of love relationships, it's no wonder that adding the difficulties of illness into the equation can create another level of complexity. As a young girl seeking love, I made many mistakes. As a young CF girl seeking love, I made many excuses. Using trial and error as my guide, I continued to make mistakes and excuses well into adulthood. There aren't many role models out there for such a situation and I fumbled desperately in the dark.

A confident person in most of life's arenas, my relationship-self never seemed to match the rest of me. When talking to boys, my focus was on saying what I thought he wanted to hear. All I cared about was getting him to like me and become my boyfriend. It never occurred to me to question whether or not I liked him!

In relationships, I was submissive and was often talked down to and told what to do. Inside, I knew that wasn't right but I couldn't bring myself to rock the boat. Deep down, somewhere along the way, I developed an unconscious belief that I had to trade bad behavior for him having to "put up" with my illness. I was often in a state of vulnerability and weakness. That state of mind led me to do things I wouldn't have done had I been true to myself. It allowed me to be in verbally abusive, long-term relationships and to hang on to those relationships out of fear of never finding better.

Many women have walked a similar path to the one I'm describing, but cystic fibrosis was a driving force behind why it was so difficult for me to change these detrimental patterns. There was unaddressed anger and sadness there, and I often looked to men to make me feel alright about my disease. That never worked! With some counseling and a determination to be loved the right way, I eventually found my way out of that confusing maze.

The Bad Boy:

In 1998, I was living in beautiful San Francisco, waiting for the call that I was high enough on the transplant list to move back home and get new lungs. There, I had met the type of man most women feel compelled to try and tame: the classic bad boy. His name was Derek and he wasn't like any other man I'd dated. He was tattooed and pierced. He rode a motorcycle. He was into the scene and knew all the cool places to go in the city. He had a shady past filled with drugs and other disconcerting choices. Somehow, that was all made right by his devotion and unexpected sweetness. I fell hard.

We dated for about a year, all the while my health was deteriorating. When I got the news that it was time to move back East to wait for my transplant he was very supportive. He owned his own business and arranged to take long leaves of absence every few months. He was going to stay with me and be there when I was healthy and back on my feet.

Derek came to visit me once. After that, the strange phone calls began. We argued and I cried. He wasn't making much sense and I couldn't quite figure out what was happening. Eventually it came out that he'd found someone new. He finally broke up with me. Well, sort of—it was a messy break with lots of phone calls and wavering. My heart was broken and I made a fool of myself trying to keep this man in my life.

All the signs had been there, had I chosen to read them. When I stopped being able to go out dancing he wondered how he could be with a girl who couldn't "give him what he needed." He was an ex-drug addict who had replaced cocaine with a girlfriend. That girlfriend happened to be me but I was easily exchangeable. When he traded me in for a newer model, it made sense but it hurt like hell.

I felt abandoned. I was in, perhaps, the scariest, most vulnerable position of my lifetime, and I'd been left behind. Worse than that, I felt ashamed. I blamed his decision to flee on my weakness. Worse still, I felt his behavior was justified. I'd been dumped by someone I loved and felt like I deserved it.

When I look back, I feel sad for that devastated girl who cried herself to sleep when she should have been saving her energies for the awesome journey that lay ahead. I feel sad for the girl that let a man make her feel invalid because of an illness beyond her control.

After the transplant, Derek came back. He wanted to move to the East Coast and "make it work." Apparently, things weren't going well with his current female obsession and he was back on drugs.

I laughed and said "Too little, too late." There was surprisingly little satisfaction in knowing he still had feelings for me. His actions and words had caused me so much pain, there was nothing that could right that wrong. I never spoke to him again.

By Myself:

After Derek, I had friends and family, but I lacked that one special person with whom I could curl up and tell my inner most thoughts. I never lost the desire to have this person and went on some pretty desperate and pathetic dates hoping to find the one.

I dreamt of the man who would hold my hand as I cried and said I didn't know how I could do this anymore. I longed for the one who would help me when I was sick and love me for who I was. I daydreamed about looking into his eyes as I drifted off to sleep before the transplant and awoke to find him by my bed afterwards.

What I learned: an oxygen tank can put a damper on dating. I never met anyone who could handle where I was in my life. I doubt I was really in a place to start a relationship anyway. All I knew was that I was lonely and wanted the comfort of a lover's arms.

I went into surgery without staring into anyone's eyes and awoke to find only my wonderful family and friends. Along the way, I found out I could give myself most of the things I was craving from a man. I learned to comfort myself. I began to understand what it meant to love myself and "be whole" without a partner. I never stopped wanting to find true love, but I did discover a self-love that allowed me to feel much less alone. I began thinking of myself as my own best friend. I know now that my loneliness served a great purpose and has made me capable of being a full person in a relationship.

Mismatch:

When I was diagnosed with chronic rejection, I'd been dating Pete for a few months. Neither of us really knew what chronic rejection meant so we blindly continued on. We'd been together about a year when we reached that place many couples do: move forward or break up. Perhaps because of my bulldozer-like charm, we chose to move forward and *move in*. I packed my things and we found a cute apartment in his town. To complicate things, the day we moved in, an oxygen tank was delivered and I became dependent on tanks and tubes twenty-four hours a day.

Over the next year, my health continued to fail and our relationship crumbled from the inside out. Had circumstances been different, it's doubtful we would have stayed together. We so rarely saw eye-to-eye and had a hard time talking through our differences. To his credit, Pete never left. He never ran from his terminally ill girlfriend, no matter how poorly we were getting along. As for me, I felt trapped in my unhappy relationship, tied down by my own illness. Where could I go in that state? It was either stay with Pete or move in with my parents. At thirty, moving back to my parents' home would have been equally difficult.

To deal with the situation, we resorted to staunch pragmatism. We made deals about everything. He had a schedule of when he could do the things that drove me crazy and I had my schedule for things that drove him crazy. We had a list of topics that were off-limits. We designed ways to fight that would honor my physical limitations. Our coping mechanisms were quite intricate.

I don't mean to say there was no love there. I respected Pete for his ability to stand steady in the storm. He admired my courage in the face of death. We loved each other but we weren't meant to be together. Had I been healthy, our relationship would've never lasted so long.

In the end, he was with me through the second transplant and the following six months. Because of his willingness to stick around, I felt I owed it to him to see if we could make it work. I imagine he felt that he'd invested so much he wanted to see if things could turn around now that I was well. I was tormented by the thought of breaking up with someone who had been so loyal.

In the end, I moved back to my original town and he stayed behind. I'll always be grateful for all that Pete did for me. I'll also always remember what it felt like to be sick in an unhappy relationship. Just because he stays with you doesn't mean he's the one. With my health, I don't have the luxury of dating people who aren't a perfect match. Someday, I'll get sick again and I want the one by my side to lift me up, not tie me down.

The One:

In my early twenties, I had followed some self-help advice and written a list of the qualities I wanted in a mate. Over the years, I revised and rewrote this list. After Pete, I threw my list away. I decided my dream man was just that, a dream. I broke down my childish fantasies and let go of my secret fairytale wishes. It was time to face reality: nobody would ever meet my specifications.

When I met Jacob, it was just another date. We'd met online and he had interesting things to say, but, then again, so did the last few guys I met. The crazy guy, the married guy and the weird guy all sounded good in cyberspace. I was becoming numb to the whole process and when I entered the wine bar where we were to meet, I expected nothing.

The conversation flowed easily and we quickly bypassed the small talk. It seemed as though our perspectives meshed on every topic and I was amazed at his ability to articulate his ideas. By the end of the night, I felt as though I'd known him for years. I was giddy with wine and good conversation, but patiently waited for the skeletons to come climbing out of his closet.

On our next date, a few days later, he told me about all the research he'd done on CF and transplant. He knew more than I did about some things! While normally I'd wait to talk about all the unhappy truths of my health and early death, he asked me questions that proved he really wanted to know the deal. We hadn't been together long before we'd gone into deep and uncomfortable waters, exploring how we'd handle saying goodbye. I was very impressed with his bravery and openness.

Jacob restored my faith in fairy-tales. Every cliché written about true love applies to us. We knew right away we'd found something special. We wasted no time entwining our lives. He's in no way in denial about my situation, but it inspires us to love harder every day. We know we don't have a lifetime, but what we have is worth it.

What I Know Now:

As a person living with illness, the road to love was often confusing and discouraging. I have the battle scars from years and years of bad choices and faulty perspectives. Now, after consciously working to change my patterns, I've found what I always hoped but never truly believed was possible. I have the happiest and healthiest relationship that any human being could hope for, with or without illness. All I can do now is talk honestly about all the things I wish someone had told me when I was searching for answers to the tough questions.

I've made myself a list of the things I Wish I Knew A Long Time Ago. They seem simple, but they really are key.

Pre-Dating Homework:

It's essential before you begin dating to clearly establish a strong foundation of self-love and appreciation. Sadly, it's easy for some girls (and boys) to see themselves as damaged goods, and, therefore, be willing to do things in relationships or overlook major character flaws they wouldn't if they didn't have an illness.

The first step in doing this is to uncover the difference between your mind, your body and your soul. We so often find our self-esteem in the clothes we wear or how pretty we feel, but it's important to go deeper to discover what's valuable about you beyond the physical. Once you're able to make that differentiation, you can explore, on a much deeper level, who you are and what you believe about life. When you can truly see yourself as the amazing person you are, you'll be able to begin the search for a healthy relationship.

Dating:

There are so many questions that come up when you first start dating a new person. Things like, "When should I tell him about my illness?" and "What kind of reaction will he have?" can distract you from getting to know someone. The answers to these questions need to be explored in your homework so you can enter into the dating world with a plan. You have to figure out where you stand on these important issues before you go on the date. Trying to sort out when you should tell someone about your physical problems in the back of your mind won't work; you won't be engaged in the moment and will miss getting to know the person in front of you. If you think of these things ahead of time, you'll have a game plan and can feel more confident.

In general, when you're on a date, it's essential to find techniques to help you maintain your level head and not get caught up in the need to impress. Pretend like it's a job interview and you're the employer! There's only one position available as your partner, so be discriminating and choose wisely!

Getting Serious:

When you have an illness, falling in love can feel bittersweet. Amidst the excitement and joy come the questions: "How will we handle it when I get sick?" "Will he stay with me when I'm in need?" and "Can I or should I have children?"

Facing the sad parts of your reality head-on is key to having a strong relationship. If you can't talk about the hard things, there'll be trouble down the road. As the person with the illness, it's your responsibility to educate and initiate dialogue about your disease process. It's your partner's responsibility to take it seriously and look within themselves to see if they're up for the challenges ahead. If your relationship is going to work, you'll both need to feel safe and comfortable in talking about your true feelings at every turn. While facing illness is difficult, it can enhance a relationship with the right partner because you'll be keenly aware of how precious your time together is.

The burning question for many single and chronically ill people is: "Can I have the relationship of my dreams despite my illness?" My answer is yes. There's someone out there who will love you enough to feel that a short time together is better than no time at all. Is your life more complicated because of your illness? Yes, but you have the opportunity to embrace your challenges and enrich your life and your love.

Anatomy of a Migraine

I woke up yesterday with a migraine. I'm familiar with the feeling and knew right away what to do. I took nausea and headache medicine and sat very still, hoping it would pass on by. This was my first migraine after having gotten the stomach surgery that prevents me from actually being able to vomit. I was dreading this day because I didn't know how things would go considering my average migraine causes me to throw up five to fifteen times. I hoped I'd caught it in time but I didn't.

I began to retch and sweat profusely. My heart pounded in my ears. After what seemed like days, the retching subsided and I began the evaluation process. Do I need to go to the hospital? Should I call Jacob at work and ask him to come home? If I'm patient will it subside? Even though my shift doesn't start for hours should I call work and tell them I won't be in today?

I made a deal with myself. I decided to wait and see if I had another bout of nausea and retching, and, if so, I'd call Jacob and ask him to come home. Minutes later I went through another round and called Jacob immediately after. As soon as I hung up the phone I was met with guilt and doubt. Was this bad enough that I needed to ask him to leave his job and come home? Should I have waited longer to see if I could get by on my own? What could he do for me anyway? Was I being a baby calling him?

Jacob got home minutes later, just in time for another round of retching. We couldn't communicate at that point and I was unable to fill him in on what was going on and what medications I'd taken. He sat with me and waited for it to be over. Once again, I was hot and sweaty and he got me a cold rag for my head. He rubbed my neck and kept the dogs away from my face. He called my work and told them I wouldn't be in that day. I felt very weak and light-headed so I asked him to help me to the bathroom. I was so unsteady on my feet I doubt I could have made it on my own.

Perhaps because I was unable to have the relief that comes with vomiting, my body started to shake uncontrollably. Jacob helped me lie down and covered me with many blankets. He then took out my dog who'd been asking me to go out prior to his arrival home. When he was gone I began to think I needed to go to the hospital. I craved the IV medications that would take away my nausea and my head pain. I decided to wait it out a little longer.

When Jacob came back, I felt so safe knowing he was there to take care of me I fell asleep. My body was exhausted. I woke up a few more times to retch and was relieved to have Jacob there to hold my hand and wipe my brow. Eventually, I slept without the need to wake up and retch. The worst of it had passed and all that was left was a headache. I knew I couldn't move around much or the migraine might regain its strength. Jacob got me some applesauce and water. I was okay and he could return to work.

Before he left, I thanked him for coming home. He said he didn't feel like he did anything to help me. I imagine from his perspective his actions were small. Getting a cold cloth and shooing away the dogs probably doesn't feel like the work of a hero. But it is.

His presence made me feel secure in knowing that if things got worse he could take me to the ER. Taking out my whining dog was something I couldn't have done and, had I tried, would have certainly caused another round of retching. Wiping my brow was incredibly soothing when I felt as though I was on fire. Holding his hand made me feel loved and reminded me I was human, not just a ball of pain and misery. He took hours away from work and contributed so much in my moment of need. I could never explain how incorrect he was when he said that he didn't do anything.

Anyone who sits with a person in a time like this one, a time of incredible discomfort, is a hero in my eyes. Whether you're a parent, a spouse or a nurse, you'll never be more needed in your life. While you may not be scaling a burning building, your energies will never be more appreciated.

Thank you, Jacob, for being there for me yesterday. Thank you, Mom and Dad, for being there many migraines before I met Jacob. Thank you to all the heroes out there who sit by and wipe the forehead of someone they love with a cold cloth.

A Letter to My Beloved

To My Dearest Jacob,

I was talking to a friend today and she was telling me about a mutual acquaintance who recently started dating a woman with a serious heart defect. Her life is hanging in the balance. My gut reaction was to ask, "Why is he with her?" It seemed almost masochistic to become involved with a woman who would soon be dead.

As soon as the words fell from my tongue, I was struck with panic. How could I, of all people, say such a thing? For just one fleeting moment, I saw myself through your eyes.

You fell in love with a woman who, relatively speaking, will soon be dead.

I've been living with illness for so long that I've become immune to some of its horrors. It was easy for me to put those scary parts aside and focus on the beauty of our connection. From my perspective, our love was simply too powerful to walk away from. I was fully immersed in the romantic ideal of true love and understood only a portion of the gravity of your position. But, in the moment when I saw it in other people's lives, I was able to appreciate the choice you had to make: Love with loss or walk away. Many would have chosen to walk away. You chose to stay and walk into the unknown realm of uncertain health and a precarious future.

In the years we've been together, you've provided me with a sturdy platform on which to stand. I've been able to reach for things that would have been impossibilities without the foundation of our relationship. You've given me unwavering love and treated me with a kindness I always thought was reserved for characters in fairy tales. You challenge my intellect while respecting my individuality. You hold my hand while helping me to my feet so I may walk on my own. You don't judge me; you're always on my side. You're my perfection.

When I think of you as the man who is with the woman who will soon be dead, it makes me sob. You deserve a relationship built for a lifetime of happiness, not just a sample. You deserve all of the strength, insight and kindness you've given me. You deserve forever. It just doesn't seem fair. Why should you get the short end of the stick?

Sometimes I simply don't feel worthy. What have I done to deserve such an extraordinary man? The only explanation that makes any sense is that God's given you to me, and me to you. I don't know why and I don't know how. I do know that to second guess it would be foolish. The only smart option is to cherish it, and I'll do that until the day I die.

You're my everything. It's such a helpless feeling to know that you'll lose me someday and I can't protect you from that grief. I can only hope we continue to use my illness as a constant reminder to treasure each day we have together. I can only pray that the life we share today is worth any pain the future may hold.

I love you.

Fight or Surrender?

I see it in so many ways and so many situations around me: the fight for survival. When I watch my friend, who is in failing health, sign up for an invasive experimental surgery, I ask myself if I'd put myself through that or if I'd simply call it a day. When I see owners drag very sick pets into our veterinary office time and time again, I wonder what my limits will be for treating my dog when she gets to the end of her life. There's no right answer, only the question.

The Fine Line:

When you work in a veterinary hospital, death comes wrapped in a unique package. With the possibility of euthanasia, end of life issues are complicated by the opportunity of choice. Owners and doctors collaborate on when they believe the animal has had enough and often opt to put them to sleep. Within this opportunity of choice lies a spectrum. On one side you'll find the owners who request euthanasia when a pet isn't even sick but is "annoying" or "aggressive." In light of this topic, this side of the scale isn't worth much consideration—and those owners' requests are denied! It's the other side of this spectrum where I find valuable scenarios worth contemplation.

From every objective standpoint, it was pretty likely Casey was dying. She was a very old dog who hadn't eaten in at least a week. The owners continually brought her in to address her appetite, with little success. She could barely walk and, at times, didn't have the energy to lift her head off of the floor. Time's passing didn't seem to calm the panic in her owners' hearts and we received many calls with requests for us to see Casey on an emergency basis. Despite the fact that everything Casey was experiencing was perfectly normal for a pet at the end of life, Casey's owners never considered the option of surrender.

After many visits and many treatments with little to no effectiveness, the doctors recommended an ultrasound. The owners agreed and Casey's ultrasound was done on a Tuesday afternoon. The test showed that Casey was riddled with cancer. She had tumors in many different areas of her body and one had begun to perforate her bowel. Upon looking at the images, there was no reason to question why Casey had been feeling so badly and, in fact, she was getting along quite well given her physical state.

Because Casey's owners had been caring for this very sick girl for over a week, and because they were so dedicated to her, I had fully expected them to take her home and spend at least one more day with her. Much to my surprise, as soon as they heard the news about the ultrasound, they chose to euthanize her immediately. It struck me that, before they knew what her insides looked like, they had no intention of slowing the fight for her life. Once they had the new information, they surrendered with no hesitation. Casey was just as sick before the ultrasound than she was after, and yet something had dramatically changed within her owners.

Casey was put to sleep and went very peacefully. The owners felt good about their decision. I certainly never doubted they made the right choice. It was, however, an interesting example of the fine line between fight and surrender.

Another Doggie Tail … er … Tale:

Scrappy—a small black and white dog—was brought into the veterinary clinic with a terrifying wound. His owner was a wonderful person who ran a very successful dog rescue organization. Apparently, for whatever reason, a group of her rescue dogs chose to gang up on poor Scrappy and attacked him quite brutally.

Scrappy had a wound on his back hip and leg that was so deep and large a person could put their fist inside it. He underwent an operation on his leg nearly every day for weeks. The veterinarians worked diligently with medicine and surgery to pull the wound together so it could close up. During this time, Scrappy's cries could be heard throughout the hospital. He was in great discomfort as well as being disoriented by the pain medications. It was heart wrenching.

After weeks of great effort, the doctors came to the conclusion that they could not save Scrappy's leg. The wound was not healing and they were worried the prolonged exposure could cause a systematic infection. They advised the owner to schedule a surgery for amputation.

Scrappy's owner refused. There was something inside her that knew Scrappy would be okay. Against medical advice, she took Scrappy home that night while many of the staff members shook their head with worry. We didn't see Scrappy for months after they left.

One day, during a staff meeting, Scrappy came in for a visit. Everyone gasped as they watched Scrappy prance around the room on four legs with barely a hint of a scar. He was happy and healthy. His owner had been right.

Sometimes, there is something inside of us that knows that it is not time to surrender. Sometimes, there is an indescribable knowledge that the doctor's prognosis doesn't apply. There is a fine line here between denial and the true knowing. In Scrappy's case, he was lucky to have a mom who knew in her heart he was going to be fine and had the strength to follow her own intuition.

What I Know Now:

When I watch some people clinging to threads of possibility for one more day on earth, I wish they could just surrender and let go of their attachment to living. Sometimes the attachment is more painful than the dying.

On the other side, there are plenty of people who have gone against their doctor's orders only to be alive and well many years after they "should" have been dead.

The only thing I know for sure is that you can never know what you'll do until you're actually in the situation. I had proclaimed on more than one occasion that I would never have another transplant. The sicker I got, the weaker this conviction became until I'd completely changed my mind. If I'd simply surrendered in 2003, I never would have gotten a second transplant and I'd have missed out on so many wonderful things. I'm glad I kept fighting.

We all have our notions of when it's time to fight and when it's time to wave the white flag. In our culture, there's a strong emphasis put on the value of fighting. In fact, when someone dies, we often say that they "lost their battle" with their disease. I don't know where that fine line between battle and surrender falls, but I do know that there's a time when giving in grants the most peace. Please don't ever tell me someone "lost their battle" to a disease. This isn't a war and there's no one to blame. Instead, appreciate when someone knows it's time to stop fighting and let life's journey draw to a close.

The question of fight or surrender will always remain just that, a question. Simply knowing there's an option for both, however, is invaluable.

Splitting the Rails

When the call came that I'd be given a chance for a second lung transplant, my reaction wasn't one that most people would expect. I was in a state of pure distress. I'd been planning my death for months and months. I'd said goodbye to so many of the people I loved. I was ready, no *excited*, for the day I'd leave here and see what waits for us on the other side. This news that I may have a chance at life threw a real wrench into the works.

To make it more complicated, there was absolutely no way to know if I'd actually make it to the transplant. This meant that what had gone from a definite—I'd die in the coming months—had gone to a complete unknown. I might get the surgery and live or I might die before any organs became available. It was about a fifty-fifty chance. This put me in a very uncomfortable position and I felt lost. I didn't know what to hope for anymore. I didn't know how to pray. I didn't know if I should continue to eat all the junk food I wanted—one of the best parts about dying—or go back to a healthier diet. I didn't know if I should stop buying the "skinny sick" clothes and wait for the day when I'd put on a few pounds to do some shopping. My concerns ranged from serious spiritual dilemmas to the mundane. I was confused. I called this feeling "splitting the rails."

I know many people face this in many different ways. When people have cancer and begin chemo, there's no way to know if it will work, and whether they will be healthy again or if it won't and the cancer will take over. When people prepare for major surgeries, they know they have a chance of the body being fixed or the body collapsing under the weight of such extensive measures. In so many different ways modern medicine brings us into the dilemma of the unknown future.

Finding peace with this situation was a difficult thing to do. I actually found myself wishing I'd never had the opportunity for another transplant. Planning my death was so much easier than planning for life and death simultaneously.

I had made my peace with the end and now I had to make my peace with a new beginning. The only way to do this was to love both of my options equally.

I had to plan for both possibilities equally, as well. I continued to plan my funeral and say my last words. At the same time, I dreamed about all the things I'd do once I was well. The image I used was that I was packing two suitcases for two destinations. One was in the cold North east, one was in sunny California. I had no idea where my bags would end up; I wouldn't know until I was boarding the plane. All I knew was they were both possible and they each required their own wardrobes. The tricky part wasn't being attached to either destination.

It took work and many tears, but I finally found myself in a place where I was thrilled with both options. I had both bags packed and waited for my tickets to arrive. This time, obviously, my ticket was for another trip to the OR. Looking back, I can see this was the greatest lesson in balance I could have ever received.

A Letter to Death

A letter written during a healthy time, after my second transplant

Dear Death,

I think I was born being uncomfortable with you. Growing up, the thought of a loved one dying filled me with cold panic and I was unable to allow those thoughts for any length of time.

When I got to be around ten, I started to understand the severity of my disease. As a ploy for attention, I'd proudly announce to my classmates that I wouldn't live into my twenties. There was a part of me that enjoyed seeing them squirm with discomfort; it was a confirmation that nobody I knew was comfortable with this topic. My proclamations were light years from my heart. I was so disconnected from the emotional truth that I shut down until high school.

I grew sicker as I grew into my teens, and spent my first weeks in a hospital around the age of twelve. There was a boy down the hall who was eleven, and he also had CF. I knew he was sicker than me because they moved him into my room to be closer to the nurses' station and kicked me to the end of the hall. One night, I saw his parents leaving, crying. That familiar cold chill went through me and I assumed that you'd taken him. Unfortunately, I was right.

I cried for him and cried even more for me. This was a boy I had never known, but we had the same disease, he was one year younger than me, and he was dead. You didn't make sense.

My uncle died not long after this event, and I remember the feeling of complete terror and helplessness as we greeted my grieving aunt and cousins. I wanted to smile and pretend we were having a pleasant family reunion, but their tears foiled those plans. I wanted to avoid the topic of my uncle entirely. I wanted to hide until the sadness around me was over. Instead, all I could do was sit in a room of grieving loved ones, half in shock and half sick to my stomach.

At thirteen, my fear of my own death was still abstract, but palpable. I began to act out in dark teenager kinds of ways. I dressed in black and wrote somber poetry about the meaninglessness of life. I drank and smoked with my friends. The smoking especially felt like a true empowerment and a screw-you to this disease and to you. I'd always seen the disease as separate from myself, and, in this case, that proved to be a great disservice to my own health.

It was many, many years later, as an adult, that I found myself face to face with you. I had to take two passes at the dying thing before I could move aside my fear and denial long enough to embrace what was happening. With time and a weakened body, I grew unafraid of your truth and welcomed your gifts.

I could write pages about the freedom that comes from accepting you as a part of life. I could write books about the beauty of dying and how it can transform your entire foundation. At least I'd like to think that I could. But the feelings of peace that I've experienced are memories now. I can only explain what I remember. I can only tell you that what should have been the worst part of my life is that part that I look back on most fondly. I can see the bitter beauty and complexity within my own experiences and the tales of those around me. I can only wish that telling my story will help others understand why a big piece of me looks forward to the dying I have to do in my future.

Thank you for everything,

Tiffany

Pockets of Grief

Often, when someone is in the middle of a trauma, be it illness or otherwise, there's not enough time, energy or perspective to process the relative emotions. For the sake of survival and sanity, they're pushed down, at least to some degree, and not addressed. Where do those emotions go? I think most people assume they simply dissipate, like smoke into the air. In fact, emotions are energy, and, as the first law of thermodynamics tells us, energy can't be created or destroyed. So what happens when we're unable to feel our feelings? In my experience, they wait until they have an opportunity, and then pop up, often at very unexpected moments.

Embarrassing Flood:

A year after my second transplant, I was taking a class a friend was teaching. It was a group of spiritually minded individuals who met once a week to learn about different spiritual principles and practices. One evening, my friend started talking about the Buddhist practice of Ton Glen. This was a meditation I used on nearly a daily basis when I was at my most ill and in a great amount of discomfort or pain. She told the class it was a meditation to increase compassion for other people and gave the details on how to practice it.

My own Ton Glen meditation had changed a little, from the way I'd been taught to a more customized version. I raised my hand and began to tell the group about the way I visualized and used this practice. (As a side note, I've put the meditation at the bottom of this chapter.)

When I began speaking, I wasn't filled with emotion other than the excitement I felt about telling the group about my experience. A few sentences into my explanation, however, it was as though I'd been hit by a bolt of emotional lightning. Suddenly, I was there, in all of the moments of suffering in which I used Ton Glen. I was in all of the moments simultaneously and the emotion was overwhelming. I began to cry, aware my tears would seem out of place within the context of what I was saying.

I felt self-conscious and willed for the tears to stop. They did no such thing. The emotion continued to build until I was sobbing and unable to catch my breath. I was confused by my own feelings and apologized for the mysterious outburst. No matter how hard I tried, I couldn't hold back this flood. I eventually had to stop telling my story altogether and continued to weep for another few hours. It was the next day before I was able to understand what had happened. I'd stumbled into a pocket of unexpressed grief.

Unfinished Business:

In 2007, I was invited to my class's ten-year college reunion. It was a weekend consisting of many events. The first was a Q-and-A with the current students in which my class of thirty answered questions about what they'd been doing since graduation. Following that were events in which we mingled with the faculty in various venues and over different themed buffets. The culmination was a big party at one of the graduate's homes; everyone and anyone was invited to attend.

While it was wonderful to see old friends, I spent the weekend feeling as though I was on the verge of tears. In everything I did, I was riding a wave of subtle sadness I couldn't shake. As I sat and watched those around me, I felt such envy. As I talked with old professors I felt a sense of unworthiness and shame. I hadn't graduated from this school. I had to leave because my health was too poor to continue. I was placed on the lung transplant list the summer after my second year and never returned to finish my degree. I envied those framed diplomas on the wall in the homes of those around me. I felt embarrassed to be the student in the room who only finished two years. I wondered if the teachers even remembered who I was.

At the final party, I fell into a pocket of grief. All the memories and all the nostalgia swarmed around me. It was intoxicating and reminded me of how passionate I was about school back then. It reminded me of the girl who wanted nothing more than to finish this acting conservatory and live the dream of being a working actor. I was hit with the sorrow that came with having to drop out and leave this dream behind. I felt such sadness for the girl who, once again, had to give up something she loved because of her illness.

That night, on my way home, I cried for that girl.

What I Know Now:

Pockets of grief may appear when you least expect them. Often, it takes time to understand what's going on and where the emotion is coming from. Because it's emotion from the past, it can feel disjointed and unspecific. The ambiguity of this kind of emotion can make it especially confusing.

I've cried for the girl that did Ton Glen every day. I've cried for the girl who had to walk away from her passions and her dreams. I've cried for her today because I can. I now have the breath and the strength to sob for her losses. I can do today what she was unable to do so long ago. The energy of these emotions have lived within me for all of these years, and now, through my tears, the grief may be transformed.

My Version of Ton Glen:

Close your eyes and get as comfortable as you can.
Take three slow breaths.
With each breath, relax more and more.
Look within yourself and discover the place where you feel the most pain.
Picture yourself standing next to your pain. The pain may be a specific object or a blob of energy.
Pick up your pain and hold it in your hands.
Imagine walking to a bank. Enter the bank and go up to a teller.
Hand the pain to the teller and inform her that you'd like to make a deposit into the account where pain is kept.
Let the teller take the pain out of your hands.
Say to her and yourself, "I offer this pain to all who are suffering with the same kind of pain, now or any time in the future. May they suffer less because I suffered consciously today."
Now picture a person—It's probably not a person you know—suffering with the same kind of pain you're experiencing
Picture them going to that bank and making a withdrawal from that account.
Picture them being soothed, their pain lessening.
They suffered less because you suffered consciously today.
Repeat: "I offer this pain to all who are suffering with the same kind of pain, now or any time in the future. May they suffer less because I suffered consciously today."

This meditation was helpful to me on two levels. First, it allowed me to feel like I was contributing to the world, even at a time when I was unable to get off of the couch. Second, every time I did this meditation, my physical symptoms were lessened. I found great comfort in this exercise.

A Bathtub Moment

Journal entry from March, 2004

I've been working very hard to accept my fate, no matter which way the wind blows. I've found a place of equilibrium and I'm happy with my options: life or death. I guess I've stopped thinking of it as death, really ... it's more a graduation. I've exerted plenty of time and energy anticipating and preparing for both scenarios equally. It's taken a few months, but I've achieved my goal and feel proud of it.

Tonight, however, I had a moment of clarity and confession—not the Catholic kind. I was taking another long bath. That's where I do some of my best thinking and praying. I said to God, "God, I know I don't really get much of a vote on this living or dying thing. I know that it's in your hands if I stay or if I go. For what it's worth however, if I *did* have a vote, I'd like to stay. I'd like to take all of the things I've learned, all of the growing I've done, and use it to serve you. It seems a shame to me that I could have gained so much insight in the last few months only to die without being able to share it with anyone. So God, if I do get a vote, I'd like to stay."

That was the first time that I've allowed myself to choose a side. It felt good to admit what I really wanted. It felt scary to know I actually do have a preference.

On March 28, 2004, roughly one week after this moment, I had my second transplant. Since then, I've always wondered if this talk with God had anything to do with it.

When Beliefs Collide

Journal entry from July, 2003

I was raised in a very Christian home. To my parents' dismay, not all of their children fell in line with that belief system. While I have a deep spirituality, it doesn't follow all of what the Bible talks about. For example, I believe in Jesus but I don't believe in a literal, eternal hell. My parents, however, follow the word closely, and hell is a reality for them. It's for this reason that my terminal illness, coupled with my beliefs, was extremely distressing for them. They feared that once I left this earth, we might end up in different eternal residences and, therefore, they may never see me again.

This issue was very painful for them and was brought up in different ways throughout my life and my illnesses. Sometimes I felt compassion for their heartache and sometimes it made me very angry. I'd even contemplated lying to them and saying I'd done all of the things they asked me to do, just so they could have some peace. Ultimately, I was pushed to a point of such frustration I chose to confront them about this issue. My plan was to lay down strict boundaries and declare the topic of religion off-limits. I'd tell them in no uncertain terms that their feelings were their problem and they should leave me out of their religious quandaries. Luckily, before I had this bitter conversation, I decided to pray about it first.

The irony doesn't escape me that my most trusted spirit guide is Jesus. I feel very close to him individually, just not the religion of Christianity. This distinction may seem strange to some people, certainly that was so for my family, but nonetheless was where I was coming from.

When I sat down to talk with Jesus, I knew my father was on his way over to spend some time with me. Because of this, I focused my attention on talking with my dad. I asked the question "Jesus, how do I talk to my dad about my beliefs?" These are the things he told me. They simply popped into my head as a conscious thought and I wrote them down.

1. Tell him that he's confusing religion with rules. Religion isn't rules, it's love.

2. Tell him you're my child and I love you. Ask him how in the world he thinks I'd ever let anything bad happen to my child?

3. Tell him everything you've done, you've done to find love. Love of yourself, other people and love of the universe. If Buddhism and other traditions help you learn more about love, they're a good thing.

4. Tell him how you always turn to me first with your big problems.

5. Tell him that when you say you love me, you mean it—not only as a practitioner, but as someone who knows me personally.

6. Tell him to lay his burden down.

7. Tell him he'll never know how much I love you but that's all that really matters.

8. Let him think on these things. Arguments are not necessary.

Arguments were not necessary. I read these things to my father and he cried. He told me he felt sure now that I'd be okay. He was able to lift his fears and sadness and embrace the concept that, despite my "non-traditional" route, I'd found my way to heaven.

My parents and I still come from very different perspectives on God and the afterlife. What this taught me was that when religions collide, there are two ways one can handle the situation. One can fight back with the force of the ego and claim "rightness," or one can dig deeper and find the spiritual thread that connects most world religions: love and compassion. I could have gotten indignant and told my parents to back off. Perhaps that would have been acceptable, reasonable. But would it have been helpful and healing? Certainly not.

By listening to the voice inside me, I was able to draw myself closer to my religious "opponent" while maintaining my own integrity. This certainly is the ideal and I'm forever grateful that I spoke to Jesus before I spoke from judgment and anger.

Marketplace Monk

There was a time when I placed my worth on outward achievements. I had a burning desire to *do more* and leave behind an impressive resume. Many of my efforts through the years have been thwarted by illness. I never graduated college. I've never been completely financially independent. There are countless projects I've started and never finished. By many standards, my life hasn't been a success. This reality has made me feel ashamed at times, and has greatly affected my self-esteem. At other moments, it makes me feel alone in the understanding of what really matters in life.

Doing, The Meaning of Success:

After my second transplant, I was working to find my place in the world. I was interested in veterinary medicine and took a job assisting a mobile veterinarian. Things started out well but quickly deteriorated. It's my belief that once he discovered I wasn't interested in being his lover, he began to lash out and try different tactics to get rid of me. One of his tactics proved to be unbelievably effective.

For reasons unknown, he'd been angry with me all day. Out of the blue, he started interrogating me about my life. I relayed some of my history, both work and health. He drilled down harder and harder, pressing me to lay out my accomplishments. The difficult truth was that there were few that were in any way measurable. He concluded our talk with a sentence I'll never forget: "So what you're telling me is that the only thing you've been able to achieve in your life is to survive."

A cold way of putting it, but, at the time, I could only agree. I saw myself through his standards and so left his vehicle that day very broken. Out of his spite and unkindness he had spoken the words I never dared speak to myself. He'd said the thing that I always imagined people secretly thought about me: My life had been a waste. I was devastated.

He had successfully gotten me to quit working for him. It's rumored that he now has a young assistant willing to oblige him in the ways I had refused.

Being, the Meaning of Success:

When I was dying, there wasn't much left of my life. I had no job and not much of a social life. At first, I was very concerned that I wasn't contributing to the world.

In time, my perspective changed. I saw the world around me with new eyes. Watching those I love run around chasing balls in a job they hated seemed so futile. Seeing those before me hate themselves for reasons unclear to anyone else seemed tragic. Witnessing people value their money more than their souls seemed ludicrous. I was living in a different dimension in which inner peace trumped all other earthly goals.

I'd reached a level of living similar to monks in a monastery. I saw only the preciousness of life and wished others would do the same. I was no longer concerned with who I wanted to be or what I wanted to do. My purpose became to be the best human I could be and I enjoyed exploring my own internal world.

My contribution to the world, it seemed, was to *be* and what I *did* meant little to nothing.

What I Know Now:

Being ill and moving through the dying process has proved to be an extraordinary teacher on the value of *being* rather than *doing*. What I've found, however, is that there's value in living both ways.

While there was great peace in living like a monastic monk, striving only to be, that existence is hardly sustainable once one leaves the confines of the monastery walls. Once I was well again, I was back in the marketplace, working for money to live, shopping for that which I required, and living an altogether more complex daily life.

I've been tempted to find more value in the world of the monastic monk. Being removed from the trappings of materialism and a nine-to-five seems somehow more enlightened. To *be* rather than to *do*: how deep and meaningful!

However, as I walk through the marketplace I find things that I want to do to improve my world. I have things I desire to do to make an impact. Clearly, there's value in doing as well.

Success isn't easily definable. It can be found inside and out. While I'm able-bodied, I'll try to carry the lessons I learned in the monastery with me, using them to the greatest benefit of my marketplace.

About the Author

At six months old, Tiffany Christensen was diagnosed with Cystic Fibrosis. Since that diagnosis she has spent countless hours in doctor's offices and hospitals. She has lived with chronic illness, acute illness and terminal illness. In order to save her life, she has undergone two double lung transplants. Through a lifetime of difficulty, this illness warrior has emerged with clarity and insight.

Enjoying the best health of her life, Tiffany is now ready to speak! She is a workshop leader and public speaker. She has a passion for educating medical students and other health care professionals. Tiffany's mission is to empower patients and educate professionals in such a way that we will begin the medical revolution.

Tiffany lives in Chapel Hill, North Carolina with her husband and two silly dogs.

Acknowledgements

Thank you to my husband and my family for listening to me babble about this book for so long, for loving me no matter what and for supporting me while I try to make this dream take flight.

Thank you to Watts and Lizzie for being the best BFFs a girl could ever want. You've been there for me through thick and thinner and I can't thank you enough.

Thank you to my transplant buddies—Suzy, Dave, Lisa and Gabe—for your humor, courage and advice.

Thank you to my medical team for keeping me alive all these years.

Thank you to my donor families for making the painful and brave decision to save lives despite their losses.

Thank you to my bloging buddies—you guys kept me going when I was tired of writing and pumped me up when I was feeling insecure.

Thank you to all of the people I wrote about in this book—good or bad—you have made my life richer.

Sick Girl Speaks! Pop Quiz

I bet you had no idea you would be quizzed on what you've learned reading *Sick Girl Speaks!* Well, if you were paying attention, you'll remember that it's time for a medical revolution. Part of that revolution entails patients taking responsibility for their care and their own empowerment. In order to do that, there's a lot to know and learn. How do you think you'll do?

1. Being a Patient Advocate means that I or someone else:
    a. Fight with Doctors and Nurses over my care
    b. Tell the Medical Staff about my feelings often
    c. Guard over my care and make sure my needs are being met

2. True or False:
    In a hospital setting, my Primary Care Physician is in charge of my care

3. In a hospital system, rank the following levels of caregivers from 1 to 11 with 1 being the top of the ladder:
    a. Floor Attending Physician
    b. Fellow
    c. Surgeon
    d. Intern
    e. RN
    f. LPN
    g. CNA
    h. Resident
    i. Chief Resident
    j. Specialist/Attending Physician
    f. Phlebotomist

4. In a hospital setting, when I have a problem with my care, the best person to talk to is:
   a.   The Floor Attending
   b.   The Intern
   c.   My Attending

5. The first rule of advocating for my self or others is:
   a.   Always be nice
   b.   Learn and know what the proper treatments and drug schedules are
   c.   Buy the nurses candy as much as possible

6. If I have a problem such as nausea, I should:
   a.   Tell a nurse and wait for them to decide what to do
   b.   Tell my doctor and see what he says
   c.   Tell the nurse and doctor that I need a prescription for my nausea

7. When I go for a doctor visit, I should bring:
   a.   My written list of medications and dosages
   b.   A written list of my questions
   c.   A written list of any symptoms that have been bothering me
   d.   All of the above

8. If I have to make a trip to the ER, I should:
   a.   Have my doctor call ahead and let them know I am coming
   b.   Bring a written list of my medications and dosages
   c.   Write my root illness as well as my symptoms on my check-in card
   d.   All of the above

9. When it comes to being cared for by nurses and doctors, *awareness* of what medications they are giving me or my loved one, the tests they are running and the procedures they are doing is:
   a.   Not important, that's their job
   b.   Important but not necessary
   c.   Extremely important, could be a matter of life or death

10. If I need sleep in a hospital, I should:
    a. Plan to sleep all night long
    b. Take naps in between interruptions
    c. Post signs on my door with visiting hours for non-essential medical personnel

11. If I am getting my blood drawn and the phlebotomist has tried and missed my vein twice I should then:
    a. Give her my other arm so she can try there
    b. Cry and yell
    c. Tell him or her to find another phlebotomist to take over

12. Questions 10 and 11 have in common:
    a. nothing
    b. They are both situations that require Boundaries
    c. They are both examples of our inability to control our fate when we get sick

13. True or False:
    Doctors deal with death and dying all the time and so they have reached a peace that allows them to be helpful to patients who become terminally ill.

14. When it comes to my Healing, the responsibility falls on:
    a. My Doctors
    b. Myself
    c. Both a and b

15. When it comes time for a person to die, it is:
    a. Always sad and scary
    b. Often fun and exciting
    c. Possible to find great peace and inner joy

Sick Girl Speaks!
Pop Quiz Answers

1. Being a Patient Advocate means that I or someone else:
    c.   *Guard over my care and make sure my needs are being met*

2. True or False: In a hospital setting, my Primary Care Physician is in charge of my care
    False. In many cases the primary care doctor is only consulted occasionally, if at all. The person in charge of your care when you are an in-patient is the floor attending. That person may or may not be well trained in your illness. It is simply the luck of the draw.

3. In a hospital system, rank the following levels of caregivers from 1 to 11 with 1 being the top of the ladder:
    1.   *Surgeon*
    2.   *Specialist/Attending Physician*
    3.   *Floor Attending Physician*
    4.   *Fellow*
    5.   *Chief Resident*
    6.   *Resident*
    7.   *Intern*
    8.   *RN*
    9.   *LPN*
    10. *CNA*
    11. *Phlebotomist*

Are there titles in that list that you don't know much about? Find out! What does it matter? It's important to understand the hierarchy of our medical system. Chances are there will be a day when you will need to advocate for yourself or someone you love. When that day comes, you'll need to know who's in charge of who so you can knock on the right door and air your complaints.

Please note: this is by no means a complete list of the professionals you will encounter in any given hospital.

4. In a hospital setting, when I have a problem with my care, the best person to talk to is:

    c.   My Attending

    When you start squeaking that wheel, chances are the intern, resident and floor attending will be the ones to step in and try to solve a problem. Keep in mind they don't know you like your primary doctor does. When things aren't going well, don't be afraid to pass them by and call in your primary attending.

5. The first rule of advocating for my self or others is:

    b.   Learn and know what the proper treatments and drug schedules are

    Being nice and buying the staff candy is a great idea but the best way to getting good care is to know enough that you can communicate intelligently as well as be able to stop someone from making a mistake.

6. If I have a problem such as nausea, I should:

    c.   Tell the nurse and doctor that I need a prescription for my nausea

    Be direct and don't wait for someone to care. Ask for what you need even if you're not completely sure what all the options are.

7. When I go for a doctor visit, I should bring:

    d.   All of the above

    Remember: pen and paper are a patient's ally. Use them wisely and you will avoid may annoyances and complications.

8. If I have to make a trip to the ER, I should:

    d.   All of the above

    This is one example of approaching health care strategically—know the ways to make it work for you!

9. When it comes to being cared for by nurses and doctors, *awareness* of what medications they are giving me or my loved one, the tests they are running and the procedures they are doing is:

    c.   Extremely important, could be a matter of life or death

Medical mistakes happen every day. Decrease your chances this happening to you by knowing what should happen and watching to make sure that everything is done correctly.

10. If I need sleep in a hospital, I should:
    c.   *Post signs on my door with visiting hours for non-essential medical personnel*
        "Sleeping in the hospital" is often a contradiction in terms. Do what you can to get as much healing rest as possible.

11. If I am getting my blood drawn and the phlebotomist has tried and missed my vein twice I should then:
    c.   *Tell him or her to find another phlebotomist to take over*
        This is my rule and you can decide what your personal limits are. The point is, don't let your body be unnecessarily damaged just for the sake of keeping quiet and not hurting somebody's feelings.

12. Questions 10 and 11 have in common:
    b.   *They are both situations that require Boundaries*

13. True or False: Doctors deal with death and dying all the time and so they have reached a peace that allows them to be helpful to patients who become terminally ill.
    False! Because of their training, many doctors see death as a failure. Don't let their disappointment prevent you from finding peace with your mortality.

14. When it comes to my Healing, the responsibility falls on:
    b.   *Myself*
        Medicating is a doctor's job—healing is a patient's job. Medicate the body and heal the spirit. Healing can be achieved no matter what the physical result turns out to be.

15. When it comes time for a person to die, it is:
    c.   *Possible to find great peace and inner joy*
        We all will have to mourn the losses of what can no longer be, but once the grief has subsided happiness is an option. There are many opportunities of illness that one can explore.

978-0-595-91611-5
0-595-91611-2